D0042587

Praise for *Looking Out for Number Two*

"A candidly written, humorous, scientifically-backed poo bible. This is an illuminating look into every parent's secret obsession—their baby's poo!—and serves as a perfect baby shower gift for new parents. I am thankful, both as a mom and pediatrician, for Dr. Vartabedian's sound advice and expertise."

> —Wendy Sue Swanson, MD, author of *Mama Doc Medicine* and founder of *Seattle Mama Doc*

"Parenthood is, unquestionably, a busy—and messy—business! While you may not have dedicated much time or thought in your pre-parenting days to the topics covered in this book, the bottom line is that you will now. And as you take advantage of Dr. Vartabedian's highly informed, practical advice, and insights about all things related to 'number two,' you're sure to find yourself thanking Dr. Vartabedian for also looking out for you!"

> —Laura Jana, MD, pediatrician and author of
> *The Toddler Brain: Nurture the Skills Today That Will Shape Your Child's Tomorrow*

"In clear, entertaining language, Dr. Vartebedian takes a bottom-to-top approach not just to poo but also to many critical aspects of child care, from childbirth to feeding, and even burping. I talk to parents all day long about feeding, burping, spitting, constipation, and diarrhea, and I found myself taking notes to share in my own practice. This book will quickly become a classic for new parents."

—David L. Hill, MD, author of *Dad to Dad: Parenting Like a Pro*

"Dr. Vartabedian has a way of taking the most complicated of medical issues and explaining them so that everyone can understand. He does this with such a wonderful sense of humor that this book is a delight to read. Both doctors and parents alike will be helped by this book. I highly recommend *Looking Out for Number Two* and hope that it is read by everyone. They will not only enjoy it immensely, but will also be optimally informed."

—William J. Klish, MD, Professor Emeritus of Pediatrics, Baylor College of Medicine

Looking Out for Number Two

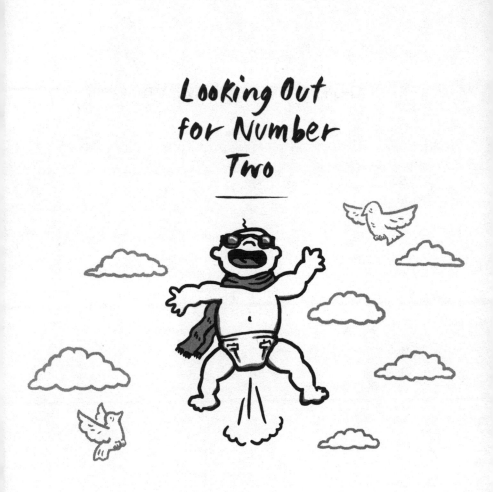

Looking Out for Number Two

A Slightly Irreverent Guide to Poo, Gas, and Other Things That Come Out of Your Baby

BRYAN VARTABEDIAN, MD

HARPER WAVE

An Imprint of HarperCollinsPublishers

This book contains advice and information relating to health care. It should be used to supplement rather than replace the advice of your doctor or another trained health professional. If you know or suspect you have a health problem, it is recommended that you seek your physician's advice before embarking on any medical program or treatment. All efforts have been made to ensure the accuracy of the information contained in this book as of the date of publication. This publisher and the author disclaim liability for any medical outcomes that may occur as a result of applying the methods suggested in this book.

FIRST EDITION

Designed by Jamie Kerner

Illustrations by Zach Harris of birdsandkings.com

Library of Congress Cataloging-in-Publication Data has been applied for.

ISBN 978-0-06-246436-1 (pbk.)

17 18 19 20 21   LSC   10 9 8 7 6 5 4 3 2 1

For Bill Klish

*Like many other women, I could not understand why
every man who changed a diaper has felt impelled,
in recent years, to write a book about it.*

—BARBARA EHRENREICH

Contents

10. GUT REACTIONS | ALLERGY, INTOLERANCE, AND THINGS THAT GO BUMP INSIDE YOUR BABY   241

11. FARTS, COLIC, AND OTHER THINGS THAT MAKE NOISE   273

12. PROBIOTICS AND YOUR BABY'S HEALTH   297

Introduction

I AM THE POO WHISPERER

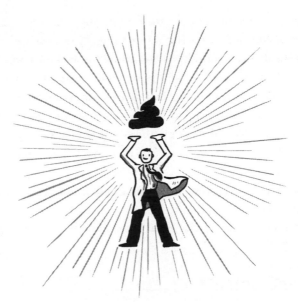

MOST PEDIATRICIANS LISTEN TO A PARENT'S STORY AND OFFER A DIAGnosis; I look at a diaper and tell the parent their baby's story. What repulses others has become my medium.

While some see a heavy, wet, rolled-up diaper as the end of something, I see it as just the beginning. If the eyes are the window to the soul, a full, fragrant diaper is the lens into a baby's biologic destiny. As you'll learn in *Looking Out for Number Two*, what happens in the deepest, darkest crevices of the bowel shapes a growing baby's future.

Dramatic? Maybe not. Read on and you'll see that there's a story unfolding around what your baby makes.

WHY A BOOK ON POO?

Let's face it: babies don't seem to do a lot. They eat, sleep, and poo. So when it comes to knowing when something's up, we measure what they eat, watch how they sleep, and look at their poo.

And when it comes to their poo, a lot is going on down there. You can see it, you'll probably feel it, and you'll definitely smell it. Poo can tell you many things about a baby's general health.

But we don't think enough about poo and what we can learn from it. The subject is cut short in most parenting books. I want to change that.

What you have in your hands is a field guide to the stuff that comes out of your baby. It's the owner's manual they never gave you in the nursery. Think of it as "what to expect when they're pooping."

WHY POO IS IMPORTANT

Traditionally, there's been a war on poo. It's the brunt of our jokes and the last thing we consider when it comes to raising happy, immunologically robust babies. But while it was long thought of as something to just wipe and flush, it turns out that what fills your baby's diaper serves an important role in shaping your baby's developing immune system.

A baby's gut is the breeding ground of the babybiome, a massive population of bacteria that are in constant communication with the immune system. And as the home of 70 percent of a baby's immune system, the gut is the body's biggest organ when it comes to making sense of the world. Everything that goes through your baby's tummy is "seen" by her immune system and creates a type of immunologic experience or wisdom, as we'll see in the coming pages. How we seed, feed, and fuel the gut early on can have a critical impact on a baby's lifelong health.

And while we're shifting our perspective on the poo front, we should consider a related area that has traditionally been an afterthought for parents: feeding and nutrition in babies. Milk, be it from the bottle or breast, is typically thought of as something to keep a baby fat and happy, a simple substrate for sustenance and satisfaction. But like poo, the things we use to fuel a baby can make or break the way a body and brain grow and react to the world. Changes in the types of protein, for example, or the presence or absence of certain bacteria are critical factors in shaping lifelong health.

So what we give babies and what babies give back are important indicators of health. Unfortunately, so much of this amazing information on babies and bowels has been restricted to research articles and the minds of experts. That's where *Looking Out for Number Two* comes in. My goals are threefold: To translate this material in a way that makes it applicable to you as a parent. To popularize and define the connection between the gut and the body and the bigger world into which a baby is born. And to get parents talking and thinking about the enteric brain (that's the nervous system in the gut, and, yes, that's a real thing), the fourth trimester of gut development (the first three months of life), and the reality of baby poo as a living, breathing organ.

Number Two is more than a book . . . it's a movement.

HOW'S HER POO?

Most health professionals begin conversations about health in babies with predictable questions about development, feeding, or sleeping. These are the metrics that have traditionally defined the well-being of a baby. When I open up a conversation about a baby, I say, "Tell me about her poo." Sure, it's an awkward question when visiting with friends over dinner, but it's a timely and important launching point in a medical context, given what we know about the gut and its miraculous work. What goes on inside a baby and what a baby leaves behind in her diaper tell so much about her well-being. And we've only begun to scratch, or wipe, the surface.

I'VE SEEN MORE POO THAN YOU

Looking Out for Number Two is loaded with the latest research, but a lot of it has been shaped by my experience as well. For the last twenty years it's been my job to understand and think about babies from the inside out. I'm a pediatric gastroenterologist at Texas Children's Hospital, the largest children's hospital in America. I've seen a lot of babies, and I've studied, smelled, and driven endoscopes straight through the stuff that comes out of them. I hope my comfort and passion about all things digestive will be reflected in the pages ahead, and that the knowledge I've gained will help put you at ease with the various diaper patties generated by your little bundle of joy.

YOU DON'T NEED THE *NEW ENGLAND JOURNAL OF MEDICINE* TO SHOW YOU HOW TO WIPE YOUR BABY'S BUM

Because some of what you'll find here represents the patterns I've seen and learned in over two decades as a doctor, not all of it is supported by journal articles or committees of discerning old men. And that's fine. Much of what we do in the care and handling of babies is based on practical wisdom.

I have full respect for those colleagues who work tirelessly to advance the margins of science and digestive health. But my goal here is to create a user-friendly compilation of translated science and care. *Number Two* is intended to serve as a practical guide to the inner workings of the baby. Science meets sensibility in this book, and it's delivered in a way that's informative, entertaining, and practical. It doesn't claim to be comprehensive, but at the end of the day I hope it will spark curiosity over something that young parents would have otherwise overlooked.

HOW THIS BOOK IS ORGANIZED

The layout of this book is simple. The first part covers what goes into your baby and the second part covers what comes out of your baby. While you could argue that I've misled you by selling a book on poo that's really only half a book on poo, the truth is that you can't understand elimination without a nod to nutrition. If you're obsessed with poo and poo alone, jump to part two.

Otherwise, feel free to just poke around. While the front-to-back narrative is laid out as a logical sequence of approachable physiology and fascinating diaper tricks, you can also just thumb through to discover some really interesting things happening inside your baby.

To make for easy navigation, the two parts of *Looking Out for Number Two* are organized into interesting bits of information under compelling subheadings. While the subheadings should clearly convey the information in a given section, I can neither confirm nor deny that many also contain poo-related puns. Consider yourself warned.

SOME HOUSEKEEPING

Following are a few things to keep in mind as you read or thumb through the book.

YOUR MILEAGE MAY VARY

No two babies are alike. Whenever I drop the "mileage may vary" comment in the pages ahead, it means that things may work out a little differently for your baby. Babies don't read. And they certainly don't read medical textbooks. When we try to apply one set of rules to something as crazy and varied as poo, gas, and burping, we're bound to wind up someplace bad.

TALKING TO YOUR DOCTOR

Parents and doctors are talking less and less these days. I wish that weren't the case, but pediatricians are under ever-growing pressure to see more patients. The time that we would normally take to sit back, cross our legs, and ponder things like stool velocity or the bigger meaning of various shades of neon-green poo is sadly decreasing. While I still ponder these issues, your provider may not—so as a parent you need to be increasingly empowered and informed.

TRUST YOURSELF—YOU KNOW MORE THAN YOU THINK YOU DO

While parenting books and media have traditionally delegated all issues and questions on baby health to the infinite wisdom of the pediatrician, times have changed. Rather than being simply followers of the pediatrician, we as parents are now partners in the care of our children. *Looking Out for Number Two* respects your sovereignty as a parent to gather information, become an expert, and make decisions about the future health of your baby.

Over my years as a physician writer, I have peppered my work with the timeless "talk to your doctor" disclaimer. You'll find that here as well, but I've come to recognize that parents are smarter than we give them credit for. The famed twentieth-century pediatrician Benjamin Spock was known for telling parents to trust themselves. This is solid advice and more relevant now than ever.

YOU STILL NEED TO PARTNER WITH AN AMAZING PEDIATRICIAN

Though the office visit may feel like forty-five seconds, you need access to a trusted partner in raising your children. If you're unhappy with your doctor, vote with your feet and find someone who meets your needs as a human and parent. A parent-pediatrician relationship is like a friendship or marriage. They work for weird reasons and we all need something different. Or as my old partner used to say, "There's an ass for every seat." This is true when it comes to finding a great doctor.

ULTIMATELY, *NUMBER TWO* IS PORN FOR STOOL GAZERS

One of my most indelible memories as a pediatric gastroenterologist was the mother who hauled a trash bag full of soiled diapers to my office. Not a diaper-pail-sized or tissue-basket-sized bag, but a Texas-sized trash bag normally used to line a fifty-five-gallon drum or haul grass clippings. For two months this woman had catalogued and saved every diaper. Date, time, consistency, color, odor, and the absence or presence of visible blood was all noted compulsively with a black Sharpie on the outside of each diaper before she taped them shut and froze them, all in anticipation of her daughter's appointment.

Filthy diapers cryogenically immortalized for my expert review.

Call me negligent, but on the day of their visit I didn't inspect a single frozen diaper. My goal was instead to complete the visit and get the family out of my office before the bag defrosted in the sweltering Houston heat. As it turns out, this child's diagnosis was made quite comfortably from her medical history and subsequent fresh stool samples.

In another case, a CPA-turned-stay-at-home-mother made repeated visits to my office with "stool portfolios" consisting of beautifully crafted 3-D pie charts and tables representing her baby's bowel actions.

Truth in a pediatrician's office can be stranger than fiction.

WHAT'S A STOOL GAZER?

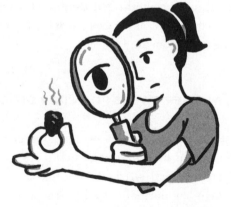

As odd as these stories may sound, they showcase an evolving parental preoccupation with diaper cakes. This is a new subvariant of helicopter parents hell-bent on the compulsive, archival recording of their baby's every movement.

They are the stool gazers.

Compulsively attendant to the shape, size, and shade of their baby's doogie, they read the best and worst into everything that appears in the diaper. Stool gazers are tenacious in trying to understand what it all means and how it relates to their child's ultimate viability for Princeton.

STOOL-GAZING: PATHOLOGIC PREOCCUPATION OR PROTECTIVE INSTINCT?

So how abnormal are these parents who carry spreadsheets detailing their child's every deed? Probably no more so than other parents whose fixation involves other organs or aspects of development.

As anyone who has ever been involved with raising a child knows, concerns over speech, growth, and behavior are the rule rather than the exception. And when a mother seeks the reassurance of a subspecialist to evaluate her daughter's speech delay, we think nothing of it. It's just that these worries seem less bizarre (and aren't nearly as amusing) when compared to those of a stool gazer sharing stories of parental angst.

But parental anxiety is considered a good thing by most—whether over stools or stuttering. Parents who are on their toes have a tendency to keep their children safe.

DIGITAL DIAPERS

As time has passed, stool gazers have become empowered with digital tools that have afforded real-time sharing and distribution of poo images. Beyond the occasional PowerPoint and PDF, poo has come my way by e-mail and text. The analog gazer has given way to a new type of digital crap compulsion.

I am aware that I may be contributing to the growing population of caregivers who are obsessed with what their babies create. And the publication of *Looking Out for Number Two* will not stem the rising tide of this emerging parental element; in fact, it may create more waves.

But waves can be good. An informed parent is an empowered, effective parent. When you know when to worry and when to chill, you'll be in a better place to care for your baby and seek expert care when needed. As your baby grows, you will become the expert on her patterns and habits. And what she creates in her diaper, how often she creates it, and even the odor of her creations will shape a pattern that uniquely defines your baby and her state of health. Remember, it's not just poo—it's a powerful piece of your baby's biologic destiny right there in your hands.

So let's go look for number two—or at least read about it.

YOU MAY BE A STOOL GAZER IF . . .

- Have you ever taken a picture of a diaper?
- Have you ever used digital or social technology to

transmit or seek social input on the appearance of a diaper sausage?

- Have you ever created a table, graph, spreadsheet, PowerPoint presentation, or document of any kind centered on your baby's bowel habits?
- Have you ever awoken in the middle of the night thinking about something that came out of your baby's butt?
- Have you ever manually dissected, divided, or explored your baby's poo?

If you answered yes to any of the above questions, you may qualify as a stool gazer. Congratulations and welcome to this one-of-a-kind fraternity.

THE BOTTOM LINE

After a career spent on the operating end of the growing digestive system, I've seen it all. I've smelled it all. And it's precisely this practical poo wisdom that I bring to *Looking Out for Number Two*. I hope you enjoy the read, and I would love your feedback. Find me on Twitter at @Doctor_V and join the discussion under the hashtag #numbertwo.

PART I

WHAT GOES IN

Your Baby from the Inside Out

AFTER A BABY'S MILK DISAPPEARS, WE DON'T GIVE IT MUCH THOUGHT until it reappears on the other end. While your baby may seem like something of a black box, what happens between when milk goes in and when it comes out is huge. The transformation of milk into poo is the result of a perfectly tuned system of nutrient and fluid extraction. A lot more is going on in there than you think.

Here are some things to keep in mind about the magic of your baby's intestinal tract:

1. **It's the ultimate source of nutrition.** That is . . . after the placenta. Before birth the placenta gives your baby all the nutrients she needs. After delivery, the gut takes center stage to replace what your placenta was doing.
2. **It's part of the immune system.** The gut plays a key role in the development of a healthy immune system. In fact, most of a baby's immune cells are in her intestines.
3. **It's a hormone factory.** It may sound surprising, but the process of digestion is under heavy hormonal control. Depending

on what your baby eats, the tummy hormones released will vary. Gut hormones shape things like hunger, fullness, and how hard the gallbladder squeezes.

4. **It holds on to fluids and minerals.** The intestines are key to holding on to liquid to meet a baby's basic fluid needs.

5. **It's home to the microbiome.** As we'll learn, the bugs found within the intestinal tract play a key role in helping a baby adapt to a world full of foreign things.

6. **It has its own brain.** There may be some truth to the accusation of having your brains in your arse. The intestines are home to a vast network of nerves rivaling those found in even the spinal cord. This enteric brain, as it's called, is critical to digestion and the elimination of the stuff we don't need.

7. **It's a work in progress.** Your baby's gut goes through several months of growth and development as it adjusts to the new outside world and all its nutrients.

A little housekeeping before we get too deep into this. Throughout *Number Two* you'll hear me use the term *gut*. When I say *gut*, I'm referring to the big long tube that runs from your baby's mouth to her bum. It's the whole system, the tubular space where digestion and absorption of food happens from top to bottom. Another term I'll use for this important tube is the *intestinal tract*. Gut is just easier since I don't have to type as much.

THE FOURTH TRIMESTER OF BABY GUT DEVELOPMENT

Pediatricians through the years have referred to the months after birth as the fourth trimester of development. That's the period of time after a baby comes down the pipe when she adjusts, adapts, and grows. Your baby's intestinal tract goes through its own fourth

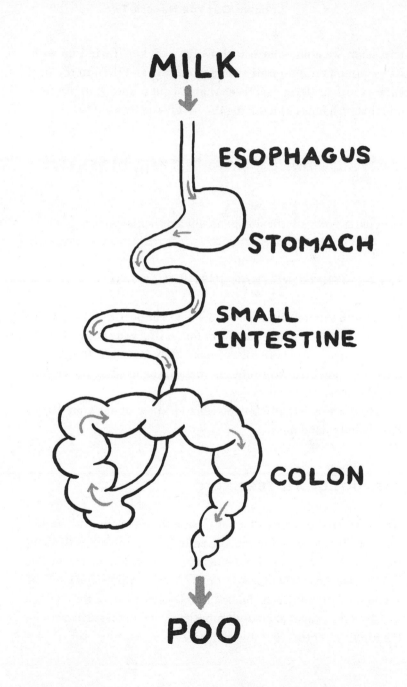

trimester; what she's born with is not what she'll wind up with. As we jump here into your baby's plumbing and then in the next chapter into bacteria, you'll see that the gut is a work in progress and that it changes a lot during the first few months of life.

BABY PLUMBING | MAPPING THE DIGESTIVE TRACT

LET'S DRILL DOWN on what happens when milk disappears.

THE MOUTH: MORE THAN JUST A MILK HOLE

The mouth is more than just a place to connect to a breast. It's not only the critical starting point for getting your baby what she needs to grow, it's where digestion actually kicks off. It's also the home of some primitive reflexes that can be used to amaze your friends and amuse your in-laws.

Here are a few things you should know about your baby's mouth and what it does.

THE ROOT OF ALL FEEDING

If you tweak the corner of a baby's mouth or cheeks with an object, they'll react with the **rooting reflex**. With this reflex the baby turns in the direction of the object and opens his or her mouth. This allows the infant to zero in on the nearest nipple and latch on. When my son did this he looked like Jaws moving in for a kill. It usually goes away at about four months of age. Babies still grab for the nipple after that, but this reflexive *rooting* is gone.

SUCK THIS

Once they latch on, babies launch into the **sucking reflex**. What happens here is that once something is inside your baby's mouth, sucking movements begin. As your milk drops into her mouth, her tongue pushes it to the back for swallowing. And while you won't be able to notice it, your baby's breathing stops for just about one second while swallowing.

The sucking reflex disappears around four months as well. Of course, babies still suck after four months—it's just not an automatic reflex. They suck and swallow because they want to eat.

IT'S THE EXTRUSION, STUPID

A baby's mouth is designed to suck and swallow and only to suck and swallow. If your two-year-old son tries to feed his new sister a Lego block, that block will likely get pushed out. Your baby is smarter than that . . . or at least her reflexes are smarter than that. The **extrusion reflex** is a natural protective mechanism that keeps out the stuff she's not able to swallow yet. It normally dries up around four to six months of age. We'll learn more on this pesky little protective mechanism when we start solids in Chapter 4.

DON'T GAG ME WITH A SPOON

Closely related to but not to be confused with the extrusion reflex is the **gag reflex**. This familiar reflex kicks into gear when something makes it past the first line of defense of the extrusion reflex—like when a spoon or a piece of solid food is placed far back in the mouth. The trigger for a gag will vary by your baby's age. In new babies, it is triggered in the midtongue. As babies get older, this trigger area moves farther back in the throat.

The gag reflex is one of the key reasons for delaying the introduction of solid foods until four to six months of age. Like these other baby mouth tricks, it goes away at four months, but it is retained on some level to keep us safe as we get older.

So A BABY'S MOUTH IS MORE INTERESTING THAN YOU MIGHT HAVE thought. Here are a few more fun facts, beyond the reflexes.

CAN BABIES TASTE ANYTHING?

Babies can discriminate a small variety of taste sensations from the first few hours of life. After birth, infants appear to be able to distinguish between sweet, sour, and bitter. But your baby actually starts tasting things around sixteen weeks of development in the womb. They can taste amniotic fluid, which, believe it or not, reflects what you eat. This passive baby exposure to tastes continues after delivery through the magic of breast milk.

And yes, your baby will be able to discern one formula from another. For example, hypoallergenic formula has a very distinct road-kill flavor when compared to a cow's milk-based infant formula. Across brands, however, your baby will have a hard time telling formulas in the same class (cow's milk-based, soy, hypoallergenic) apart. While even you can appreciate the pungent odor of hypoallergenic formulas, the taste can actually impact how your baby feeds in the event that she needs a formula change for milk protein allergy. More on this when we discuss allergy in Chapter 10.

BABY'S BREATH

One thing that you may notice about your baby's mouth is the fact that her breath doesn't have much of an odor. Why no morning breath? Breath odor is driven by the bacteria in the mouth, which are limited in a young baby. Babies also don't have teeth to trap rotten food. And breast-fed babies receive a heaping dose of living cells called *phagocytes* that chew odor-causing bacteria.

SPIT AS THE FIRST DIGESTIVE JUICE

Beyond sucking and selectively eliminating rogue Lego blocks, the mouth is actually a full-blown digestive organ in babies. It makes **lingual lipase** and **salivary amylase,** enzymes that start the process of breaking down fats and carbs long before milk ever hits the stomach. This is key because the digestive enzymes from the baby pancreas and liver are slow to get going after birth.

THE SWALLOWING TUBE: MORE THAN JUST A LAUN-DRY CHUTE

After milk is swallowed, it's carried through the swallowing tube to the stomach.

The swallowing tube, or esophagus, is about eight to ten centimeters (three to four inches) at birth and doubles in length during the first two to three years of life. Parents like to think of the esophagus as a laundry chute for milk. But it's far more involved than that. Consider this: There are nearly as many nerves in the esophagus as there are in the spinal cord. All those nerves coordinate the sequential and rhythmic squeezing of muscles in wildly different patterns depending on whether a baby is ingesting milk, squishy baby food, or her first taste of diced chicken.

As milk makes its way down the pipe, the *lower esophageal sphincter* (the valve that connects the esophagus to the stomach) opens to let milk in. As we'll see in Chapter 6, the esophagus can be a big source of pain in babies thanks to acid reflux. The lower esophageal sphincter and its tendency to open and close on a whim can be part of that problem.

THE LENGTH OF A BABY'S DIGESTIVE TRACT AT BIRTH

At birth, the intestinal tract (small intestine and colon) measures approximately 360 centimeters in length (that's about twelve feet) and doubles between birth and the pre-teen years.

THE STOMACH: WHERE MILK LANDS

Milk lands in the stomach, and acid begins to work where your baby's saliva left off. Our kids come into the world ready and rarin' to digest with adult acid levels (a metal-burning pH that's below a pH of 4.). The stomach also makes a handful of hormones and enzymes that do important things for digestion.

WHAT THE STOMACH HOLDS AND WHY IT GROWS

The baby tummy starts small but expands quickly:

STOMACH CAPACITY

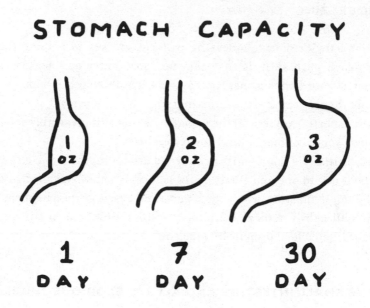

Day 1: The stomach holds approximately one ounce.
Day 7: The stomach holds approximately two ounces.
Day 30: The stomach holds approximately three ounces.

That's a pretty steep curve. The baby stomach doesn't get big quickly because of *growth* but because of *stretching*. The stomach is made of the same muscle as a woman's uterus, so it can stretch to fit whatever happens to get inside of it (like triplets, or a whole lot of milk). The progressive stretch of the baby stomach is key because it has to expand to hold the stuff that makes babies grow. And it's the stretch and collapse of the stomach that causes the release of the stomach hormones that tell your baby when to cry for food and when to stop feeding.

SQUEEZING

Your baby's stomach-squeezing patterns are key to helping the stomach push stuff downstream for more nutrient absorption. Just as your baby's arms, legs, and speech develop over time, so does the squeezing of the intestinal tract. It's slow to start, though, which partly explains all the urped milk that will invariably show up on your shoulder . . . and down your back.

Initially, a baby's milk is churned around in the stomach for about one to one and a half hours before it is slowly pushed into the small intestine, where the biggest and best digestion happens. As your baby's stomach matures, it will evolve into an organized, coordinated food propulsion machine.

THE SMALL INTESTINE AND ALL ITS GLORIOUS JUICES

Once milk leaves the stomach, it goes into the small intestine, which is effectively a black hole of digestion and nutrient absorption. More than a hole, the small intestine is actually a tube that measures about ten feet at birth. It will grow to measure about nineteen feet by the time your baby goes off to college. The lining of the small intestine is covered with little seaweed-like fingers that stick out and increase the area for absorbing things.

Inside the gut, bile from the liver and enzymatic juices from the pancreas conspire to help fats and proteins break down. Specialized transporters in the lining of the gut move sugars, special fats, and broken-down protein from the inside of the gut to the bloodstream, where they create a critical source of energy and the building blocks for growing organs.

THE COLON

After all the key nutrients have been sucked from what your baby's sucked, the remainder lands in the colon. This is a big, wide, slow organ, and it represents the final pathway to creating what you find in the diaper. The colon is about two feet long in a baby, and there's a stretched part at the end called the rectum. Poo is stored in the colon before it goes into the diaper. After a meal, waves of muscle contraction move through the colon and push poo along. When the wave hits the rectum, poo is pushed along reflexively, thereby creating a glorious diaper patty.

As the ultimate poo organ, the colon doesn't get a whole lot of respect. But you should take a moment to be thankful that your baby has a colon for a few reasons:

- **Water salvage.** One of the key roles of the colon is to hold on to water that doesn't get absorbed in the small intestine.
- **Energy salvage.** During the fourth trimester, babies aren't up to snuff when it comes to absorbing nutrients. The colon has a unique mechanism for capturing the energy that the small intestine misses. Bacteria in the colon take unabsorbed carbohydrates and make them into compounds called *short-chain fatty acids*. These are then more easily absorbed and used as a key source of energy for babies.
- **Home of the biome.** Finally, and as we'll learn in the chapter ahead, the colon is the safe haven to a critical majority of bacteria that take up housekeeping inside your baby.

The Babybiome | The Power of the Creatures Within

B Y NOW YOU'VE COME TO SEE THAT A BABY'S BOWELS ARE PRETTY AMAZing. But what's more amazing than your baby's ability to digest fat, protein, and nutrients is what you find inside the gut: bugs, and lots of 'em. Trillions, in fact. But what are they doing there, and why are they important?

BUGS AND THE FOURTH TRIMESTER: ZERO TO ONE HUNDRED TRILLION IN A FEW DAYS

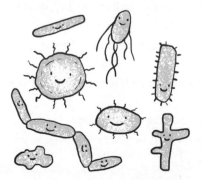

How babies evolve after birth is mind-boggling when it comes to their bacteria.

When your baby comes down the chute, she enters the world essentially free and clear of any living bacteria. But within a few days she goes from having zero organisms in her body to about one hundred trillion. That's more bacteria than stars in the Milky Way. After a few days of life, bacteria will ultimately outnumber your baby's body cells by about ten to one.

MICROBE MAJORITY

> *The human baby is made of ten trillion cells and is ultimately home to some one hundred trillion organisms. It makes you wonder who's in charge?*

As it turns out, your baby and her various warm, moist spaces make the perfect home for bacteria. While it's inconceivable for most young parents to imagine, babies are covered with bacteria—top to bottom. Most are in the gut, but some also take up housekeeping in the nose, airway, skin, ears, and other select cracks and crevices.

These bacteria will ultimately make up a specific population of organisms that will stay with your baby and play a lifelong role in her health. Think of your baby as her own little evolving eco-system. All these bugs within us are called our *microbiota* (the term *microbiome* is used when describing all the genetic stuff inside of those bugs). I like to refer to what's in your baby as the *babybiome*. It's a little different from what's in you, and it may even be more important.

Since every bacteria has genetic material, your baby's micro-biome is her second set of genes—these are unique to your little bundle of joy and bring her a novel set of physiologic powers. So beyond the genes that come from our parents are the genes that we pick up early in life—our bacterial genes.

The surface of the intestinal tract measures in at a whopping three hundred square meters, most of which are covered with organisms. Within the gut we find bacteria in the mouth, stomach, small intestine, and colon. The numbers of bugs increase as we go farther down the intestinal tract. The biggest population of bacteria are in the colon, where they make up most of your baby's poo.

The idea that our babies have bugs up and down their gut is significant because these unicellular creatures have a really important job. It's not a matter of chance that bacteria settle and multiply by the trillions inside your baby—it's a matter of design. Just the right exposures at just the right time shape your baby's bacterial population in just the right way. Usually when we talk about bacteria, we like to talk about fighting them. But it turns out that the bugs your baby grows have the ability to determine health or disease later in life.

Babies and bugs live together in happy harmony, with no shouting or fighting between them.

GOOD BACTERIA AND BAD BACTERIA

Bacteria tend to get a lot of bad press and freak parents out. That's because, for the better part of the twentieth century, all discussion about bacteria was made with warlike terms. We did battle with pathogens, the bacteria that can cause disease. Fighting the stuff that caused infection was a crusade of sorts—and it's true that pathogens are dangerous, especially for babies. So we're programmed to think of bacteria as bad bugs, and we take them very seriously.

But we need to remember that in addition to the bad bacteria, there's also plenty of good bacteria. In fact, the majority of our body is housed with innocent bacteria that do great things for us and our babies. And it's important that we separate the bad bugs from those that work on our behalf.

YOU CAN'T CHOOSE YOUR BABY'S GENES, BUT YOU CAN CHANGE HER BACTERIA

You can think of what's in your baby's microbiome as her second genome. In fact, the total DNA of these bugs is more than your baby's DNA. While this sounds like biologic trivia, it's important for this reason: *we can't change the genetic material that comes baked into our own cells, but we can change the bacteria (and the bacterial genetic material) that live within our children.*

Read that sentence again because it's really important.

You've likely heard that saying that you can't change what you're born with. But the good news is that the things we do, or don't do, as parents can shape our baby's bugs and, in turn, set her up for a long healthy life with healthy bugs and a happy, balanced immune system.

MORE THAN A HUMAN BUCKET OF BACTERIA, YOUR BABY IS FULLY LOADED WITH FUNGUS

Just to keep things interesting, there's more crawling up and in your baby than bacteria. There are also hundreds of viruses that make up her enteric **virome** as well as a resident population of fungi that compose her personal **mycobiome**. So while you may feel pretty safe with that little sanitizer tube hanging off your diaper bag, the reality is that we live in a filthy world and your baby is literally covered and filled with living organisms.

But that's probably a good thing. And that's how we need to change our thinking. What's on our babies or in our babies plays a big role in helping them process what they'll ultimately face in a harsh, dirty world. While that sounds kind of scary, you really should feel empowered. Because the bugs our babies get are partially in our control.

POO IS ON US, NOT IN US

It might be reassuring to know that the trillions of bacteria, viruses, and fungi "in" your baby's gut are actually on the outside of her body. Stay with me on this: The gut, or the tube that food passes through and poo passes out of, is not inside of the body. It is actually on the outside of the body—it's an external tube that runs through the center of your baby's body, connecting one open end to the other. Think of the lining of the gut as an extension of the skin. So by that logic, our bacteria, and our poo, is *on* us not *in* us.

MORE THAN A STINKY LOAD: NINE WAYS THE BABYBIOME MAKES FOR A HEALTHY TUMMY

All these trillions of bacteria that make up a baby's inner genome collectively do some really important things. I like to think of poo and all the hardworking bacteria in the gut as the forgotten organ. So what do all those bacteria do to qualify as an organ?

1. **Enable nutrient absorption.** Colonic bacteria are critical in the formation and absorption of vitamin B12, thiamin, riboflavin, biotin, and vitamin K.
2. **Occupy valuable real estate.** There's a limited amount of beachfront property for bacteria on the lining of the gut. So when a baby's intestinal tract is populated with bacteria that do good things, there's less room for the bacteria that do bad things (what we call *pathogens,* or—more simply—bad bugs).
3. **Make their own bug repellent (or bacteria repellent).** The good bacteria can actually produce antibiotic-like chemicals that make bad bugs uncomfortable.
4. **Make slime.** Intestinal bacteria make *mucin,* a product that lines the intestinal tract and helps serve as a protective inner coating of defensive goo.
5. **Digest the indigestibles.** Our bacteria work overtime digesting fiber and releasing nutrients for absorption by the colon. And while our bodies produce several enzymes like lactase (for lactose) and sucrase (for sucrose) for digesting carbs, the babybiome is an enzyme machine responsible for some 260 other enzymes. Bugs that can digest plant-derived carbohydrates called glycans are present in a baby's tummy before we ever think about weaning. This means that long before a baby can take food off a spoon, the gut and its residents are priming for bigger and tastier things.
6. **Tighten the lining.** Baby bugs help the cell lining of the gut stick together and keep out things that don't belong. Bacteria also stimulate cell growth, which makes for a thick, well-developed intestinal tract.
7. **Stimulate critical Immunoglobulin A (IgA).** IgA is a critical product of a baby's immune system that serves as the first line of defense in surrounding foreign invaders. Breast milk has lots of IgA. In the baby gut, bacteria help the body create IgA.

8. **"Talk" to the cell.** Intestinal organisms are in a constant dialogue with a baby's immune system in a type of buggy gossip called "cross-talk." This helps keep the immune cells on their toes and in touch with the outside (or inside) world. For example, bacteria produce substances called short-chain fatty acids (SCFAs) that influence immune cells. As it turns out, these SCFAs act as a critical link between the microbiota and the immune system by shaping and controlling the development of infection-fighting white blood cells.

9. **Colonic salvage.** Baby nutrient absorption isn't superefficient, and bacteria play a critical role in capturing calories not absorbed in young babies. This ability of the colon to *rescue* energy that might end up on a wet wipe is called *colonic salvage* and it's a key digestive phenomenon for babies.

Maybe now you'll think long and hard as you stuff that crapped-out diaper into the Diaper Genie. That's not just shit . . . it's an organ.

THE GUT-BABY BRAIN CONNECTION

As it turns out, bacteria also play a key role in behavior, and the connection between the gut and a baby's brain is a hot area of research right now. As we'll learn in Chapter 11, there are clear bacterial imbalances associated with colic. And specific probiotic strains have been shown to influence how much babies cry. We also know that the overgrowth of bacteria that produce d-lactic acid (a special metabolic product) in older children can create crazy, erratic behaviors. The details of the baby brain–gut connection are still being worked out, but it's clear that what you wrap up in a diaper may ultimately influence the way your baby thinks and behaves.

HOW THE BABYBIOME IS BUILT

EVERY BABY HAS A POO PRINT

We all have a population of bacteria that we start with in our baby-biome, and it's uniquely ours. Though it might resemble our parents' microbiome, ultimately it's a population of organisms that's ours alone.

While an infant may start life with one footprint, modifications in health, diet, and environment can change the babybiome. Our bugs have what's called *plasticity,* meaning they can change and morph as a group in response to what we eat or how often we use antibiotics. The good news is that, despite our potential as parents to mess up the babybiome with a lousy diet and too many antibiotics, we can sometimes redirect it later.

Your baby's poo print changes slowly over the first year of age. By early toddlerhood, her babybiome has evolved into a full-fledged adult microbiome. This population of bugs will follow your little bundle of joy mostly unchanged throughout the rest of her life. In fact, most folks see no change in their microbiota again until they hit their golden years, making the permanence of this poo print quite impressive.

WHERE DO BABIES GET THEIR BUGS?

As I previously mentioned, a hundred trillion bacteria take over your baby's body in the course of a few days. Once you've processed that slightly creepy reality, you may step back and wonder where these bugs are coming from—and what determines which bugs our babies get.

Essentially, the babybiome is the product of a baby's environment. A baby's bugs are shaped by how she is delivered, whom she hangs with, and how she's fed during the earliest days of life. Genetics and gestational age also play a strong role in determining the babybiome. And, as we'll see in the next section, the bugs that will ultimately shape your baby's digestive and immunologic destiny are aligning *inside of you* as a mom before your baby ever comes down the pipe.

MAMA KNOWS BEST | THE MAMABIOME AND THE BUGS OF PREGNANCY

The bugs your baby touches down with are part of a master biologic plan that begins during pregnancy. As you know, we all have our own microbiota (in mothers I like to call this the *mamabiome*). There are a lot of obvious things that change when you're pregnant, but one unexpected change is the balance of your bugs.

And, like other things, it all starts in the vagina. Early in the first trimester of pregnancy, your vaginal bacteria change dramatically. Bugs that are typically abundant become scarce, and less common strains start showing up. Generally, though, the bugs in the vagina become less diverse.

Research done by Dr. Aagaard-Tillery at Baylor College of Medicine has shown that one particular bug, *Lactobacillus johnsonii*, becomes abundant in the birth canal during pregnancy. Usually found in the gut and not the vajayjay, this bacterial strain is key to the digestion of the milk sugar lactose. Billions of lactobacilli slather your baby as she makes her way into the world; presumably, the mamabiome changes in this way to help populate a baby's gut and get her ready to digest milk.

The intestinal mamabiome undergoes some wild changes near the end of pregnancy as well. It's been reported that the bacterial profiles in the third trimester look a lot like those seen in obese people. While it isn't known *why* this may be the case, it's clear that there are significant changes in energy demand while carrying a child, and the bugs in the gut may potentially play a role in shaping how energy is used.

These changes in the maternal microbiota leading up to pregnancy provide further evidence that the microbiota functions like a bona fide organ. They also give new meaning to the idea that mother knows best.

DIRTY DELIVERIES SHAPE THE BABYBIOME

The way you deliver your baby can have a big impact on the bacteria she gets. In fact, as we'll see in a few pages, what seems like a small difference in how we birth can actually shape a baby's risk for problems later in childhood.

So how do vaginal and C-section deliveries differ with respect to babies and bugs? Consider what happens when a baby is born vaginally. During the fantastic journey through the birth canal, she's exposed to all kinds of bacteria that have been specifically modified during pregnancy.

The rectum, as you hopefully know, sits right next to the vagina. As that bulbous infant head passes down and through the vagina, and as mom bears down to create the requisite pressure for delivery, there's a big, unmentionable mess as a baby crowns. By design, nature brings babies into the world facing the mess (facedown, typically). This precarious positioning sets up your baby for a mouth full of bacteria during those first breaths, cries, and swallows. While it's hard to imagine this as a good thing, it's probably critical. A natural delivery is also more likely to result in a new mother holding her baby immediately after delivery, where skin-to-skin and skin-to-mouth transmission of bacteria occurs.

The C-section is another story. After a sterile prep in the operating room, a baby is taken from her sterile uterine environment and is received in a sterile blanket. Spirited away with a bunch of nervous people in masks, her gut becomes the product of the hospital environment and the skin flora of those who happen to have immediate, direct contact.

Because of these differences, the bacteria that your baby winds up with will likely be different depending upon how she's delivered. Babies born vaginally are more apt to harbor predominantly *Lactobacillus* species, whereas C-section babies are more likely to be colonized by a mixture of less friendly bacteria found on the skin and in hospitals, such as *Staphylococcus* and *Acinetobacter.* In general, C-section babies have biomes that are less varied than their vaginally transitioned nursery counterparts. They also (interestingly) have slightly higher rates of asthma, food allergies, and tummy infections.

And it seems that what happens in the delivery room stays in the gut: the differences in intestinal flora based on the type of delivery have been found to follow a baby up to seven years. But more important than just a different family of bugs is the impact that different flora have on the immune system. We'll talk about this shortly.

BUGGY WOMB DWELLERS

Not to throw a wrench in things, but it's also possible babies start getting their bacteria before they're ever born.

At the turn of the twentieth century, French pediatrician Henry Tissier was the first to suggest that babies were born into the world sterile. The idea has stuck ever since. And while many still consider the newborn to be a sterile creature, research from Washington University in St. Louis recently demonstrated the presence of microbes in the placenta. How these bugs end up in the placenta became the focus of gynecologist and Texas Children's Hospital researcher Kjersti Aagaard-Tillery. She went one step further by sequencing the bacterial DNA found in placentas to identify what kind of bugs they were. What her team discovered is that the mysterious womb dwellers most closely resembled the microbes from the mouth. Animal studies support that mouth bacteria have an easier time getting into the bloodstream and, in turn, setting up shop in places like the placenta.

It isn't clear that these bugs are doing any good for the growing fetus. And in fact, studies have suggested that microbes dwelling in meconium (prenatal poo) may be responsible for the premature birth of some babies.

So what does this mean if you have a baby inside of you? Probably not much. Bacteria are part of who we are and what we carry in our mouths. We can't change that. Maybe in the future we will understand more about how shifting the mamabiome impacts the blossoming fetus.

HOW YOU FEED IS WHAT YOU GET

After the method of delivery, what you choose to feed your baby is perhaps the most important determinant of the babybiome. In fact, based on what we just learned, if you can't deliver your baby vaginally, it's doubly important that you look at *how* you nourish your new baby.

The bugs found in a formula-fed baby and breast-fed baby are *entirely different*. And it may be this microflora difference that accounts for the powerful health enjoyed by breast-fed babies.

When it comes to seeding your baby with the right bugs for success, the way to start is with breast milk. Period. End of discussion.

Actually, let's keep the discussion going. . . . What is it about breast milk that makes it the secret weapon for seeding the baby bowel?

- **Breast milk comes fully loaded with bugs.** Coming in with several hundred identified organisms, breast milk is the ultimate seed of the babybiome. While there are bacteria common to most breast milk, there are variations from mama to mama and even differences depending upon what part of the world you're from.
- **Breast milk is the source of the almighty bifido.** In healthy, breast-fed infants, *Bifidobacteria* are the predominant bacteria in the digestive tract. Bifido (young, hipster researchers refer to it as "bifido," so that's what we'll do from here on out) is the golden boy of the breast-fed biome, and it's established as kingpin by about six days of age when it outnumbers other species by a factor of one thousand to one. This reign of colonic dominance lasts through the first year of life until breast milk is fully replaced with solid food.

In contrast, babies that are fed with infant formula have only one-tenth as many bifido in their gut as breast-fed babies. Instead, the artificially fed infant's bowel harbors a complex variety of microorganisms, including biologically less-friendly species such as *E. coli*.

Your baby gets her bifido from your breast milk. But what's interesting is that bifido can't survive on the surface of the breast since it's killed by air exposure. It's actually *in your breast*, specifically in the glands that make and move the milk (quantities vary from mom to mom). And it gets there by a process called reverse translocation, meaning *it moves from your gut to your breast and into your baby.* This is another example of how the bugs that are in you are the bugs that wind up in your baby.

You might be wondering why it matters whether or not your baby receives bifido, but it's actually a pretty big deal. Bifido is one of the key players believed to help the immune system develop just right. Studies have found a lack of bifido in children with food allergies. Other studies have shown a link between bifido and obesity—specifically, babies with high levels of the anointed strain had greater protection from future excess weight gain.

- **Breast milk is loaded with bacterial fertilizer.** Another reason breast milk is the perfect food for jump-starting the babybiome: it contains complex carbohydrates called oligosaccharides that can't be digested by humans. In fact, oligosaccharides are number three on the breast milk ingredient list. While your baby can't digest this nutrient, her bugs can. The oligosaccharides that you produce for your baby serve as critical fuel for the right bacteria. Think of human milk oligosaccharides as fertilizer for good bacteria like bifido.
- **Breast milk sugar is a powerful bug fuel.** Lactose is the key carbohydrate in human milk. Early on (during the first week of life), it's not entirely absorbed and actually helps cultivate populations of lactobacilli and bifido. Lactose may even create the environment that protects the neonatal gut against bad bacteria.
- **Breast milk doesn't neutralize stomach acid.** Bacteria live and die by subtle changes in their environment. By keeping the gut environment slightly acidic, the growth of less-hospitable bacteria is discouraged. So it's not that infant formula sets the stage for bad bugs, it's just that breast milk helps facilitate the cultivation of a superhealthy babybiome with just the right milieu.

Despite how definitive all this may sound, it's interesting to note that the breast milk biome is in a dynamic state of flux depending on your baby's age. For example, just after delivery your milk is rich in *Staphylococcus, Streptococcus,* and lactic acid producing bacteria. After six months of breast-feeding, milk becomes rich in oral cavity bugs. This is nature's way of prepping for solid food.

So while you may approach early feeding decisions from the perspective of convenience, the choice you make will result in a very different population of bugs inside your baby. And this difference is possibly the key to why breast-fed babies enjoy such brilliant health when compared to formula-fed babies.

But if you can't breast-feed, is there anything you can do to give your baby a leg up during the early days? Yes. But sit tight. We'll cover that in Chapter 12.

DÉJÀ POO | OR WHY YOUR BABY'S POO MAY SMELL
LIKE HER DAD'S

After delivery and feeding, whom we hang with is the next key determinant in shaping the bugs our babies get. Just think about what we do with our little bundle of joy. We hold them close, kiss them, and even stick our filthy, bacteria-laden fingers into their mouths. Whether we realize it or not, the everyday hugs and kisses do their part to seed our kids with what we've got.

This can be a good thing and a bad thing. Because ultimately it means that your baby's poo is the spawn of you. It's like déjà poo.

The frightening reality here is that your precious daughter's poo could ultimately smell like her dad's. And while the baseline criteria for modern mating was once a tall man with smarts and good looks, fecal gas patterns may soon emerge as a key element when choosing a life partner. A bold prediction, perhaps, but a relevant consideration nonetheless.

Beyond inheriting the potency of your mate's flatulence lies some bigger stuff. The idea of giving bugs to our kids is important because it gets back to the fact that our babies have a whole second genome growing inside of them—and it comes from us as parents. Just as we pass our genes on to our kids, we pass on our microbes and their associated genes as well. In fact, it would appear that the populations we harbor and transmit can shape predisposition for disease. *B. adolescentis,* for example, is more common in infants with food allergy, and there's evidence that this may be passed from parents to babies.

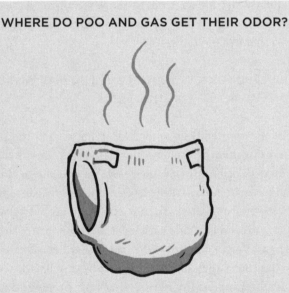

WHERE DO POO AND GAS GET THEIR ODOR?

Your baby's poo gets its odor from its bugs. More specifically, odor is a product of what your baby's bugs make. Through the process of scavenging leftover sugars and sundry bits of fiber, bacteria release gases as well as by-products called short-chain fatty acids. So depending on the unique bacterial balance your baby bears, expect an odor all her own—or maybe like yours.

And if you are blessed with the capacity to pass gas that smells like rotten eggs, understand that you may pass this skill on to your baby. The talent of generating rotten egg farts identifies you as a *methane fermenter.* That means that you harbor a population of bugs that produce a significant amount of methane gas. But don't despair. You can sleep well knowing that some 30 percent of the population produces substantial quantities of methane resulting in noxious, room-clearing flatulence just like yours. And if you've spawned methane-producing progeny, it's further evidence that the apple doesn't fall far from the tree—and that how you seed your baby's gut is the direct result of what you've got.

CUTTING-EDGE RESEARCH SHOWS THAT MOTHERS ARE LESS GROSSED OUT BY THEIR OWN BABY'S DIAPER

The good news (apparently) is that despite what your baby's diaper patties smell like, science tells us that you'll be enamored with what they create. And this, too, may be by design.

File this under crazy, but Australian researchers determined that mothers are less grossed out by the smell of their own baby's diapers when compared to other babies' diapers. In a bizarre blindfold test, mothers Down Under were forced to face ripe, wafting diapers from different babies and then rate their degree of repulsion. The study suggests that the maternal acceptance of a baby's doogie offers an evolutionary advantage in keeping the human species afloat.

But I don't recommend you try this at home, and remember that being repulsed doesn't make you a bad mom (or dad).

THE FIVE-SECOND RULE, TOE CHEWING, AND OTHER FORMS OF GUT INOCULATION

No discussion of tummy bugs would be complete without acknowledging the foul things that babies stick in their mouths.

As parents we spend the better part of early childhood working to keep our kids alive. Part of that involves keeping shit out of their mouths. Literally, in some instances. Beyond shit there are coins, pointed objects, shiny magnets, and other sundry items that look good to a crawling baby. While we compulsive parents see chewing and mouthing as potentially dangerous, it may offer kids an immunologic advantage for survival.

In fact, infantile oral exploration helps to facilitate the colonization of the gut with bacteria. It makes sense, doesn't it? Kids are learning to understand their world. While sticking things in the mouth involves tastes and textures on the lips (and temporary relief from painful teething), this may also be a calculated move to acquire bugs, and lots of 'em.

Most seasoned parents live and die by the five-second rule, and I have a theory that this rule has played a critical role in infant bowel health. For most parents, picking something off the floor comes with the innocent logic that if we can't see it, it can't hurt us . . . or our kids.

The reality is that five seconds is more than enough time for a sticky teething biscuit to be inoculated with whatever happens to have colonized your yellow lab's slobber. But this may not be such a bad thing, since children from households with dogs are subject to fewer chronic illnesses such as asthma.

In fact, maybe we should change it to the thirty-second rule. Or just eat off the floor.

PUDDING AND PROCESSED PUREES—HOW PARENTS ARE
CHANGING THEIR BABIES FROM THE INSIDE OUT

Beyond how we choose to feed our babies during the early months of life, what we do when it comes to solids definitely impacts the babybiome. One of the biggest shifts that occurs in the babybiome comes when your baby moves into solid foods. What and how you feed your baby impacts what she will grow or harbor.

To start, industrialized, highly processed foods have been shown to promote bacterial populations that look very different from those seen in people fed more natural, fiber-containing foods. And this probably isn't a good thing.

In a landmark 2015 study published in the journal *Nature,* mice that were fed emulsifiers (the chemical in processed food that makes pudding smooth) developed evidence of colitis like that seen in children with ulcerative colitis and Crohn's disease. The authors of the study concluded that the food-processing chemical given to the affected mice either (1) changed the protective mucus layer in the gut or (2) helped breed mucus-penetrating bugs.

Emulsifiers are just one of hundreds of chemicals used to make artificial food look appealing and natural. And apparently they work to make our microbiota look anything but natural.

ANTIBIOTICS—HOW BABIES LOSE THEIR BUGS

Beyond how a baby is born or fed, one of the biggest forces shaping the babybiome is antibiotics. And when I say shaping, I don't mean for the better. Despite the work you may do to ensure that your baby gets the right microbial start in life, antibiotics will level that advantage in a matter of days. Some hard-won flora, when wiped out, may take months to return—or may fail to ever repopulate the intestinal tract.

The unoccupied real estate that comes with absent bugs creates a once-in-a-lifetime opportunity for less-than-friendly bugs to set up shop. And kids who have had lots of antibiotics have less diverse flora, a situation that puts them at risk for later disease.

Antibiotics can come from places other than your neighborhood pharmacy. Your baby and her precious babybiome may be exposed to low levels of antibiotics once she moves on to solid food, as antibiotics can be found in water and some meats. Ranchers use low levels of antibiotics in their cattle—not to keep them from getting sick, but to help them gain weight. Beyond exposing your baby to antibiotic residue, this practice is breeding superbugs resistant to antibiotics. So be careful how you source your food and stick to USDA organic when possible.

THE BABYBIOME AND THE IMMUNE SYSTEM

OKAY, SO YOU'VE got a baby with trillions of bacteria in a combination all their own. There must be more to this story. Certainly these bacteria are doing more than sitting around creating unique odor patterns.

And in fact, they are. The bacteria in the intestines are in constant communication with the immune system, highlighting two of the most important elements of your baby's bugs: where they live, and who they talk to.

BACTERIAL BACK TALK

Few people realize it, but the gut is the home of a new baby's immune system. As we learned, some 70 percent of a baby's immune cells live in the gut. It's where the immune system comes to understand what's foreign and what isn't. It's where a baby learns to experience or "see" the world in an immunologic sense. So when it comes to survival in a threatening world, the gut is the center of your baby's testing ground.

While we have bacteria in our sinuses and on our skin, the gut flora are different because they're the ones in closest connection with your baby's immune system. As it turns out, those hundred trillion unique bacteria and this mass of gut-associated immune cells actually talk to one another—in fact, they talk up a storm. It's like a cocktail party where nobody's showered.

This buggy cross-talk helps the fledgling immune system understand which bacteria represent a real threat and which don't. The babybiome is critical in helping create the settings on what a baby's body should react to, both now and later in life when she becomes your much bigger baby.

Think of the gut as a training ground for a healthy immune system. The babybiome is like a personal trainer, but much cheaper and without a spray-on tan.

LEARNING HOW TO LIVE IN A CRAZY, FILTHY WORLD

Most important, the bugs that you deliver to your baby help her learn how to live in a filthy world full of crazy foreign things.

We once thought of the immune system as something that fought bugs. We now see it as something that helps us adapt to and live with the bugs around us. Without exposure to a peaceful population of bugs, a baby's immune system would never learn to tolerate foreign things. And tolerating some foreign things is critical, because most foreign bugs and things we encounter in our environment are not harmful. If your baby's body were to attack every new thing, it would be in full attack mode all the time and it wouldn't be able to direct its resources at fighting what needs to be fought.

It turns out that the immune system's ability to *tolerate* bacteria may be more important than its ability to *fight* bacteria. And this ability to coexist with a certain population of bugs and then react appropriately to a dangerous infection is a critical life skill that all babies develop during the early months.

Scientists might say that the bacteria your baby picks up and cultivates are important in suppressing inflammatory response and promoting immune tolerance. Another way to think about it is that a healthy babybiome helps our children develop a balanced and even take on the world around us.

WHAT HAPPENS IN THE GUT DOESN'T STAY IN THE GUT

While your baby's bowels are the testing ground for all things foreign, the experience doesn't end there.

As babies encounter all kinds of foreign proteins and organisms during the first year of life, the entire body benefits. Immune cells that come to the bowel to train move from the intestine throughout the body, acting as diplomatic emissaries with information and know-how about what our immune system needs. These gut-based missionaries deliver messages about what to get excited about and what to leave alone. In this way, a baby's immune system is very gut-centric and dependent upon the bacteria and foreign exposures in the gut. And what happens in the gut can impact far-reaching organs like the lungs, skin, and brain.

This is why I like to think of the gut and its resident poo as the most important organ in the body.

THE ASTHMA-BACTERIA LINK | PICK YOUR FLVR

Asthma is an example of a disease that can come from the over-reactivity of our immune system. It's a chronic inflammatory disease of the airways that can arise from some combination of environmental exposures and reaction by the immune system. It isn't clear why some people get asthma and some don't.

Asthma is a growing problem for us and our children. Three hundred million people worldwide suffer from asthma, including twenty-six million in the United States. The incidence of asthma in the States increased from 3.1 percent in 1980 to 8.4 percent in 2010, according to the U.S. Centers for Disease Control and Prevention.

While asthma has a clear genetic component, bacteria (or lack thereof) may also have the ability to lead your baby to wheeze. While it's known that children who have taken lots of antibiotics are at a higher risk for developing asthma, it's becoming clear that the absence of certain bacteria may play a role in tilting a child toward immunologic overreaction and asthma eruption.

Researchers from British Columbia have shown that children with asthma have lower-than-typical levels of four specific kinds of bacteria. These bacteria were nicknamed FLVR based on an acronym from their scientific names (*Faecalibacterium, Lachnospira, Veillonella,* and *Rothia*). This link between the absence of certain bugs and disease gives hope that we'll someday be able to predict disease based on poo patterns—or, more important, prevent or treat disease with targeted bacteria.

Or, as we'll talk about next, maybe we can prevent asthma and other diseases with the way we give birth.

HOW YOUR VAGINA CAN PREVENT FOOD ALLERGY IN YOUR BABY

While you may not have thought of the vagina as a critical organ of allergy prophylaxis, think again. It seems that how you deliver a baby can impact her risk for allergy.

Norwegian researchers studied 2,803 children and looked at their risk for developing food allergy based on how they were delivered. They studied babies born from three groups of moms:

- Women without a history of food allergy who gave birth vaginally
- Women with a history of food allergy who gave birth vaginally
- Women with a history of food allergy who gave birth via Cesarean

They followed these babies for two years and then looked for evidence of food allergies. Now hold on to your seat . . . as they report in the *Journal of Allergy and Clinical Immunology,* among mothers with a history of allergy, babies delivered by C-section had about a threefold increased risk of allergy to egg, fish, or nuts when compared to babies born by vaginal delivery.

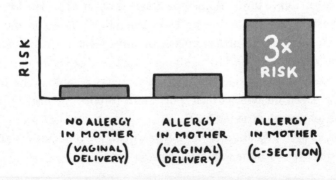

C-SECTION AND RISK FOR FOOD ALLERGY

How can that be? And why would the mode of baby delivery have anything to do with food allergies?

It seems that the poo-in-the-pie-hole situation at birth that I detailed earlier puts a baby at a distinct advantage when it comes to early colonization with bacteria. And this superearly exposure among vaginally born babies seems to create an advantage with regard to the prevention of later food allergies.

Babies born by C-section are also much more likely to suffer from asthma, type 1 diabetes, allergic rhinitis, inflammatory bowel disease, and celiac disease. This is alarming when you consider that nearly a third of U.S. deliveries are Cesarean and the number is on the rise. While it is hard to directly prove that less-than-sterile vaginal deliveries result in serious disease later in life, the association is nonetheless interesting and worth noting. The studies that have suggested an association between bug exposure and attenuated risk for disease have led to some very interesting ideas about how clean we should work to be.

THE HYGIENE HYPOTHESIS | WHY A DIRTY BABY MIGHT BE A HEALTHIER BABY

As a culture, we've become sterile crazy.

Our obsession with dirt and disinfection is officially out of control, and nervous, hovering parents aren't helping. They chase their kids with disinfectants and refuse to put them in a shopping cart unless surrounded by a personal cart canopy (true confession: I've done it myself).

We've done our part to shelter our kids from the most basic things in our world. But it may be that a lack of exposure to bacteria early in life can create more problems than we might have thought. Because when babies are sheltered from interactions with bacteria, they lose the opportunity to develop an experienced and tolerant immune system. This could potentially set them up for health problems in childhood (as we saw with C-section babies previously) or more concerning chronic diseases of adulthood.

For millions of years we coexisted with bacteria in a neighborly kind of way, each helping the other survive and thrive in our environments. But our culture of cleanliness may have disrupted the balance. The parental drive for hand sanitizer on every diaper bag and the demand for babybiome-obliterating antibiotics at every sneeze has done its part in altering the early intestinal flora, potentially at a serious cost. I'm pointing my finger at the doctors who are willing to dole out antibiotics at every nervous mother's command when there's no indication for their use, and at the growing number of sterile C-sections that are used to deliver babies. As we saw, these environmental elements affect how the microflora is established and how the immune system learns.

MICE WITHOUT MICROFLORA

Theories are a great place to start, but scientific studies are necessary to help test those theories. So what happens when animals are raised without bugs? It ain't pretty. *Gnotobiotic* animals (those born and raised in sterile environments) have sick, weak-looking intestinal tracts. And the diseases they suffer from bear a striking resemblance to what we see in kids with autoimmune disease. All signs point to the fact that bacteria may be your baby's best friend.

This idea that a clean world creates a potentially dangerous world for a child has been called the *hygiene hypothesis*. The cleaner we've become, the greater your baby's risk for things like eczema, asthma, and allergic conditions. This hypothesis was initially based on observations that being part of a big family protected against hay fever, while smaller families were thought to provide insufficient infection exposure due to fewer snot-nosed kids. And while I'm not advocating barnyard animals as house pets, parents need to recognize the critical importance of letting our kids (and their immune systems) see the world for what it is.

It's interesting to look at what happened over the second half of the twentieth century. Doctors did a terrific job of making the world a cleaner place. My medical ancestors got rid of a bunch of terrible diseases like mumps and measles. The hard work of public health professionals made the world a shinier, safer, and nicer-smelling place.

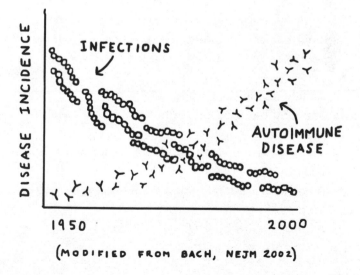

(MODIFIED FROM BACH, NEJM 2002)

But over the same period, we began to witness a rise in autoimmune diseases like diabetes, asthma, multiple sclerosis, and Crohn's disease. A likely explanation for these increases comes from the lack of exposure or experience a baby's immune system now has with bacteria in this cleaner world—because when faced with exposure to these bacteria later in life, the unprepared immune system overreacts against the body to create these terrible diseases.

This rise in autoimmune disease that happened as hygiene increased is called an *association*. It's a suggestion of a connection, but we can't say that one caused the other. But the association should be enough to cause concern and take the hygiene hypothesis ever more seriously.

WHAT'S CHANGED OVER THE LAST FIFTY YEARS?

As our world has become cleaner, what are the specific things that have led to a reduced bug exposure for our babies? Or, asking the question another way, what have we done to screw up the babybiome?

- An increase in C-sections
- Sourcing our food through a more sanitized, processed food supply
- An increase in feeding babies artificial milk (or what you might call formula)
- A decrease in our consumption of natural, fermented food
- An increasingly urban lifestyle
- An overuse of antibiotics

While modern medicine and lifestyles have done their part to make our world a safer place, all these things have reduced a baby's early exposure to bacteria and deprived the growing immune system of critical exposure and experience.

SHOULD YOU INFECT YOUR BABY TO STRENGTHEN HER IMMUNE MUSCLES?

So does this mean that you should deliberately expose your baby to people and things that will make her sick? Actually, no. The scientific view of the hygiene hypothesis has evolved over time. It seems that the exposure to a range of bugs during the first months of life is what's critical to the developing immune system. There's less evidence that recurrent infections with pathogens (that is, bad bugs and viruses) are important to boost infection immunity or prevent allergies.

So seeing and experiencing lots of things may be more important to a babybiome than getting sick a lot.

BACTERIA ARE YOUR FRIENDS

My hope is that this chapter has helped parents take a more kumbaya, hand-holding approach to bacteria than a combatant approach, and that you all are learning to see bacteria as your baby's friend rather than her enemy. Nature put bacteria in a mother's vagina, colon, and breast milk for a reason. Accept them, embrace them, and for goodness sake don't kill them unless you have to.

This is a new century with new ideas, and the bacteria your

baby comes into the world with can ensure she grows up healthy. How the babybiome develops could be a matter of life and death.

BOTTOM LINE: FOUR WAYS TO ESTABLISH A HAPPY, HEALTHY BABYBIOME

As we've learned, we can actually shape the babybiota with what we do and what we feed. Here are the top ways to help your baby develop robust microflora and a strong immune system:

- **Deliver your baby naturally.** While mothers ultimately need to do whatever is necessary in terms of type of delivery to secure the safety of them and their babies, a vaginal delivery is key to getting babies off on the right foot.
- **Breast-feed.** Do this right from the get-go. Avoid formula unless absolutely necessary.
- **Avoid processed foods.** After starting solid foods, parents should avoid processed foods and instead feed their baby natural, unprocessed foods, which will fuel the right population.
- **Use antibiotics only when necessary.** Allow the use of antibiotics only when absolutely necessary and under no other circumstances.

Milk | Power Fuel for the Fledgling Digestive Tract

No two hemispheres of any learned professor's brain are equal to two healthy mammary glands in the production of satisfactory food for infants.

—OLIVER WENDELL HOLMES

Y OU CAN'T UNDERSTAND WHAT COMES OUT OF YOUR BABY WITHOUT first understanding what goes in. And you can't talk about what goes into your baby without talking about milk.

Most of us don't pay enough attention to what we're giving our children, from the earliest decisions about breast versus bottle onward. But the decision about how to fuel your baby is probably the most important early decision you'll make about your child's health.

MILK AS MEDICINE

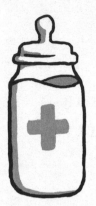 IF YOU'RE SKIMMING through *Looking Out for Number Two*, one of the most important takeaways is that milk is medicine. This idea differs from what we see in most sources of parenting information, which tend to treat all milk sources alike. It's your choice, we're told and sold. But ultimately, our babies become the choices we make.

The way we see baby nutrition has changed dramatically over the past generation. It used to be that milk and food was just something to make our babies fat and happy. It was all the same so long as nobody was crying.

But we now know that *what* and *how* we fuel our babies in the early months can set a child's lifelong health trajectory. Early feeding plays a functional role in preventing future disease. In developing countries, for example, not breast-feeding a baby can be a death sentence. In developed countries, the impact of feeding choices are more subtle but still important. Here the choice to not breast-feed can spell the difference between a healthy life and an increased risk for things like childhood allergy and autoimmune disease.

As you'll see below, what you feed is what you get.

NO MILK SHAMING

Starting from birth, babies can only receive breast milk or formula. Breast milk is the ultimate nutritional substrate for babies, since it provides precisely what a baby needs in addition to a heaping dose of immunological support. Formula represents an excellent alternative and contains all the basic ingredients for growth and development, but it should be reserved for those babies who are unable to be breast-fed. This could include circumstances such as when a mother can't safely breast-feed (due to medications, for example) or when a baby's medical situation dictates that her needs can't be met with breast milk alone (severe allergy or failure to grow properly, for example).

But while breast is best, let's get something straight: *Looking Out for Number Two* is not about milk shaming. That's the feeling of shame and maternal moral guilt that comes with the choice not to or inability to breast-feed, and that's not the goal here. And the good news is that for those moms who don't or can't feed their children naturally, there are things that we can do as parents to improve the odds that what we feed our babies shapes them for a great future. These details are scattered throughout *Looking Out for Number Two*, specifically in the chapters on allergy and probiotics.

BREAST MILK AS THE ULTIMATE POWER FUEL

The American Academy of Pediatrics (AAP) recommends human milk as the sole source of nutrition for healthy infants for the first six months of life and supports continued breast-feeding for at least twelve months. Let's start by focusing on what makes breast milk the ultimate fuel for the baby body.

WHAT MAKES BREAST MILK SO DARN MAGICAL?

It's important (and maybe empowering) to know that breast milk has lots of variability from woman to woman. What you create for

your baby is uniquely yours and tailored specifically for your child. And beyond the fact that this is a substrate uniquely concocted for your baby's specific needs, there are some consistent arguments for choosing the breast over bottle.

Let's boil down the ten top facts that make breast milk so worthy of worship. When I talk breast milk at cocktail parties, this is what I focus on.

BREAST MILK IS ALIVE AND BRIMMING WITH BIOACTIVE FACTORS

While you might see this as a little creepy, it's actually pretty cool: Like poo, breast milk is a living, breathing organ that sustains your baby during the fourth trimester of development. It's packed with *bioactive factors* (nonliving ingredients that impact a baby's body) that stoke a healthy gut and protect against infections. These factors include lactoferrin (a powerful prebiotic), lysozyme (a natural enzyme that breaks down bacterial walls and helps fight infections), cytokines (proteins critical for immune system communication), growth factors (natural stimulants that help the lining of the gut get thick and healthy), enzymes (natural chemicals that stimulate reactions), and nucleotides (one of the basic structural units of DNA). It's also full of infection-stopping antibodies like secretory IgA, which serve as a baby's critical first line of defense since newborns don't create their own antibodies until weeks after birth.

BREAST MILK IS DIRTY (IN A GOOD WAY)

There are over four hundred different species of bacteria that have been identified in breast milk. And as we learned in Chapter 2, these bugs are there for a very good reason. The breast-fed babybiome is totally different from the formula-fed biome, and your baby's gut can only get such a varied bacterial start with breast milk.

SHOULD YOU CLEAN YOUR BREASTS BEFORE FEEDING YOUR BABY?

Though you may be preoccupied with cleanliness as a new parent, don't clean your breasts before feeding. Your skin is a key source of the bacteria you pass on to seed your baby's growing biome.

BREAST MILK COMES WITH BUILT-IN BUG-SPECIFIC BIOFUEL

Breast milk provides not only a wide assortment of bacteria, but also the high-octane energy needed to sustain those important bugs. *Human milk oligosaccharides (HMOs)* are the third-most-abundant compound found in breast milk (after lactose and fat) and serve as a type of postfetal fertilizer for the expanding babybiome. We often refer to things in food that stimulate good bacteria as prebiotics (we'll talk more about prebiotics in the chapters ahead). Beyond pumping up the power bug *bifidibacteria,* HMOs set a baby up for the ultimate move to solid food and may even prevent bad bugs from sticking to the wall of your baby's gut.

HMOs make what we feed our babies uniquely human, since not even cows have it in their milk. While more than 100 HMOs have been identified, they are not found in most infant formulas. The most abundant human milk oligosaccharide, 2'Fucosyllactose (2'FL), was recently added to several Similac formulas. While not as potent as HMOs, other manufacturers have added nonhuman oligosaccharides to bring infant formula (and the gut bacteria of the babies who drink it) closer to that of a breast-fed baby.

BREAST MILK CHANGES AND MORPHS WITH TIME

Few parents realize this, but just like every living thing, breast milk changes and morphs with time. Not only does it change during a feed and even over the course of a day, it changes over the course of months to match the needs of your baby. Nearly every macronutrient in breast milk changes in some way during the course of lactation, with the most striking changes occurring in the balance of protein, fat, and energy. Your baby's demand for energy doubles between birth and her first birthday, and breast milk (and the amount your baby takes) meets the demand by changing and evolving in sync with her metabolic needs.

Contrast this with infant formula, where the approach is one size fits all. What babies get at week one of life is exactly what they get during month ten. Yet their nutritional needs are completely different. The good news is that the formula industry has recognized this natural wonder of evolving breast milk and is beginning to offer customizable milk options tailored to a baby's age and specific nutritional needs.

YOUR THREE MILKS

While breast milk changes during the course of a baby's first year, it also evolves quickly during the first few days of life. During the course of breast-feeding, mothers will actually make three kinds of milk:

your three

MILKS

- **Colostrum.** Ingested in teeny-tiny amounts during the first days of life (one-half ounce in the first day), this is a superrich source of protein, fat-soluble vitamins, minerals, and lifesaving bugs and antibodies. It gets its yellow color from the high concentration of carotene, a vitamin A precursor.
- **Transition milk.** This in-between milk moves in between weeks one and two, bringing *less* protein and immunoglobulins and *more* calories, fat, and milk sugar (lactose).
- **Mature milk.** Milk is mature about two weeks after birth and it carries babies through the first several months of life until food is started.

BREAST MILK PROVIDES THE RIGHT BALANCE OF PROTEIN FOR HEALTHY METABOLIC PROGRAMMING

Breast-fed babies are at a lower risk than formula-fed babies for obesity. The *early protein hypothesis* proposes that the difference in protein concentration between breast milk and infant formula could, in part, explain this discrepancy. Formula-fed babies consume up to 70 percent more protein than breast-fed babies during the first six months of life, and research has shown that increased protein intake results in increased levels of insulin-releasing amino acids. It's estimated that 13 percent of cases of childhood obesity can be explained by high protein intake in babies fed with conventional formula.

BREAST MILK OFFERS THE OPPORTUNITY FOR AN EXPANDED PALATE

When you breast-feed, what you eat is what your baby tastes. Flavors make their way through your milk to your baby's palate, resulting in early exposure to a wide variety of foods. According to a University of Illinois study, babies breast-fed for their first six months were 81 percent less likely to reject food as preschoolers and 75 percent less likely to develop food *neophobia*—that's psychological double-talk for the fear of trying new foods.

BREAST MILK AS BRAIN FUEL

Breast milk is brain food. Studies have shown that children who are breast-fed can potentially count on a few more IQ points—and, by one report, greater odds of higher income later in life! While there are a number of compounds in breast milk that may contribute to this difference, long-chain polyunsaturated fatty acids

(LCPUFAs) impart the most benefit on the brain. These magic fats are key to brain and eye development and are baked into the breast milk recipe.

BREAST-FED BABIES SUFFER FROM FEWER HEALTH PROBLEMS

According to a report from the Agency for Healthcare Research and Quality (AHRQ), breast-feeding is associated with a reduction in ear infections, gastrointestinal infections, respiratory infections, eczema, asthma, type 1 and 2 diabetes, leukemia, and even SIDS. It looks like breast milk could put me out of business!

BREAST MILK IS A SOURCE OF THE MELLOWING AGENT PROLACTIN

Breast-feeding triggers the release of *prolactin,* a happy hormone that makes mama mellow and relaxed. If raising your baby hasn't taken its toll on your nerves, it's likely that it will at some point. And you'll need all the help you can get.

BREAST MILK IS FREE AND ALWAYS AVAILABLE

Breast milk is free and doesn't require a diaper bag or cooler, just a drape (or not). By comparison, a year of infant formula will run you in the neighborhood of 1,700 U.S. dollars. Annualized over eighteen years in a conservative mutual fund instead, that could add up to one to two years of college tuition.

BREAST MILK ICE CREAM

While you won't need to look far to find peers who have used breast milk in their coffee, the passion for nature's miracle knows no limits. Recipes abound for breast milk ice cream and other savory treats, such as breast milk cupcakes with "boobycream" frosting. One Swiss master chef has made his mark with a bestselling breast milk soup. We can argue about the practical limits of its culinary capacity, but there's no argument that breast milk has a passionate following. And for the record, there is little evidence of breast milk's superpowers in adults.

ALMOST MAGICAL FORMULA

THE BENEFITS OF a mother's milk go well beyond my greatest hits list. But breast-feeding doesn't work for every mother. If you can't breast-feed, it's important to understand the why and how of formula-feeding and to know what you are putting into your baby's body.

Remember what I said a few pages back: how you choose to feed your baby is perhaps the most important choice you'll make in shaping your baby's future. Sure, not breast-feeding is a compromise, but not understanding the basics of baby milk is another compromise.

I call this section *almost* magical formula because recent advances in neonatal nutrition have created amazing options for those babies unable to receive breast milk. The formula options for mothers who can't breast-feed still do a great job of nourishing baby brains and bodies. In addition to highlighting the strengths of infant formula below, I'll help you combat the weaknesses through a better understanding of the ins and outs of these complex mixtures.

So let's talk about baby formula in a way that makes sense.

WHY IS STRAIGHT TALK ABOUT FORMULA IMPORTANT?

Breast-feeding is easy because there's not much to think about; mothers' breasts do most of the heavy lifting. For the formula-fed infant, parents need to be aware of a few things up front.

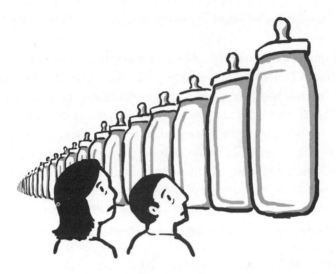

- **Infant formula is confusing.** If you go to the formula aisle in the Super-Duper Baby Superstore, you'll find a veritable plethora of formula options. I call this aisle the *Great Wall of Formula*. On the Great Wall there are a bunch of milk manufacturers, each peddling a handful of products designed for every digestive occasion. On a certain level, these options are intended to bamboozle you and pull you in by promising solutions to things that you're worrying about or that you think may be happening with your baby. Understanding your options and what your baby actually needs can be a challenge when facing this wall of choices.

- **Infant formula is expensive.** And that's why the industry wants you confused. The business that comes from the
  non-breast-feeding set drives a billion-dollar baby milk bo-
  nanza. Once you settle in to the artificial milk that you believe
  soothes, settles, calms, or quiets, you're on the hook for a year
  (or longer, as we'll see), which may represent a $2,000 com-
  mitment. You've heard of Big Pharma . . . this is Big Milk . . .
  or Big Bottle.

- **When you're uninformed, you're likely to play formula roulette.** When the promise of a formula that soothes, settles, and
  calms *isn't* met, you're likely to go back to the Great Wall to look
  for the right solution. You may indiscriminately jump from
  one formula to the next in a wild pattern of parental consumer
  behavior that I call *formula roulette,* in the hope that you'll hit
  on something that will fix your baby. But when it comes to
  nourishing your baby, hope is not a strategy and formula roulette is more likely to leave you broke and bewildered.

- **Your doctor may be confused.** If parents were more informed
  about formula, I suspect that half the confusing formulas on
  the Great Wall wouldn't survive. But the hard reality is that in
  turning to your doctor for a professionally informed decision,
  you might wind up just as confused. This is difficult to admit,
  but when it comes to training baby doctors, the area of nutrition is our big weak spot. Pediatric training has failed to keep
  doctors abreast of the escalating changes in baby nutrition.
  This isn't a criticism of my colleagues, just a reality of a world
  changing faster than most can keep up with—and something I
  hope to alleviate with *Looking Out for Number Two.*

- **Parents are increasingly taking milk matters into their
  own hands.** It used to be that feeding changes only happened on the recommendation of a pediatrician. But with
  advancing nutritional knowledge, shrinking doctor visits,

and democratized information, empowered parents have begun to take matters into their own hands. Milk beyond what the breast can deliver has become a thing of personal choice.

IT'S CALLED FORMULA TO SOUND SCIENTIFIC

Born in the days of test tubes and men with white hair in white coats, formula was given its name in the early twentieth century to deliver the promise of science, precision, and better babies. And the way infant formula is portrayed hasn't changed much. It is still promoted to parents as offering solutions to a baby's problems. While breast milk is the real formula, infant formula has been engineered to provide a reasonable alternative if a mother can't breast-feed.

FORMULA IS EASY: THERE ARE ONLY TWO TYPES YOU NEED TO THINK ABOUT

When we look at baby formula, there are only a few things that define it: protein, fat, and the calorie count per ounce. These are the core things we think about when positioning a formula.

Speaking in very general terms for the average baby, the most important ingredient that defines her formula is its *protein*. This is the element that is most likely to determine how a baby behaves . . . or misbehaves. In other words, the most common reason for changing a baby's formula is to change the protein she's being fed. When we look at formulas in this way, there are only two categories that you need to know about as a parent.

1. BASIC COW'S MILK FORMULA

This is the standard-issue stuff that you give your baby if you can't breast-feed. The protein used in standard infant formulas comes from cows (casein and/or whey), but it's broken down a wee bit and added in in just the right amount so that it's safe and nutritionally appropriate for your baby.

There are three or four major manufacturers of standard infant formula, and the basic elements of these milks are very similar since they're regulated by the FDA. The two main milks in this category are **Enfamil** and **Similac.**

Inside the category of basic cow's milk formula are formulas made of partially broken-down protein. These formulas are made with the milk protein fraction whey, which is broken down but not as much as a hypoallergenic formula. The main formula in this category is **Gerber Good Start**.

There is new evidence that the use of a formula with a partially broken-down protein might be helpful in preventing allergy symptoms (like those from atopic dermatitis, a type of eczema) in babies from families at risk. We'll drill down on this in Chapter 10.

2. HYPOALLERGENIC FORMULAS

The second category of formula that you'll need to understand from a protein perspective is the hypoallergenic category.

As you'll learn in Chapter 10, about 5 percent of babies suffer from an allergy to the milk found in standard infant formula. What we do in that case is offer a formula where the protein has been heated and treated to break it down into smaller, less immunologically threatening pieces. These smaller pieces are less likely to be recognized by your baby's gut—or, more importantly, the immune cells in her gut—which means they are less likely to provoke an allergic reaction. The same amount of protein is available in these formulas for your baby to grow, it's just delivered in a way that tricks the growing immune system.

If you're like a lot of parents, you're prone to tasting what you give your baby. Honestly, I'd pass here. These broken-down formulas stink. As it turns out, when you take a protein and digest it a bit, the loose ends of the protein chain create an odor. "Roadkill" has been the description used by some, although I can't say I've ever gotten close enough to a dead possum to confirm. Most babies don't seem to mind it, although there are exceptions.

The players here are **Nutramigen**, **Alimentum**, and **Extensive HA**. And be prepared for sticker shock, as hypoallergenic formulas will run you in the neighborhood of $350 a month for the typical four-month-old baby. For the seriously allergic baby there are super-hypoallergenic formulas where the proteins are more extensively broken down to their most basic elements. We'll cover those in Chapter 10.

WHAT HAPPENS IF YOU GIVE YOUR BABY MILK OUT OF THE CARTON?

So if we're giving our babies cow's-milk-based formula, why not just give them milk out of the carton? It's a reasonable question, but as it turns out, cow's milk is good for cows, not babies. The minerals, vitamins, and electrolytes found in cow's milk are difficult for a baby's growing kidney to process. And the amount of protein and the level of certain minerals in cow's milk is too much for a tiny gut. When babies are exposed to milk out of the carton, they may do okay in the short run but they usually experience irritation of the intestinal lining and slow bleeding with repeated exposure.

ALLERGY: THE ONLY REAL REASON TO CHANGE YOUR BABY'S FORMULA

The only hard-and-fast reason for you to jump formulas is if there's a highly suspected, or confirmed, milk protein allergy. If that's the case, you can change the protein by switching from a standard to a hypoallergenic formula.

Parents often believe that hypoallergenic formulas are easier to digest, but that is not the case. Despite the fact that the protein in these formulas is broken down a little more, we don't give them to babies to ease the burden of digestion. We use them when their little immune systems overreact to protein.

And despite the vague promises of neonatal bliss found on the labels of some infant formula, there are no dietary solutions for colic. However, babies with inexplicable fussiness may be struggling with true allergy, so a trial of a hypoallergenic formula is a reasonable and standard intervention if you or your pediatrician truly suspect a cow's milk allergy.

Milk allergy is a pretty big deal for parents, so we'll dive a little deeper in Chapter 10.

FORMULA ROULETTE: THE OTHER "REASON" TO CHANGE YOUR BABY'S FORMULA

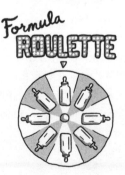

If you're not switching because of a suspected allergy, jumping formulas won't get you very far. Because within a category of formula (standard or hypoallergenic) there's little variation between the products. When parents jump from product to product it becomes formula roulette, a game of chance where parents who don't know better desperately try to leverage the only thing they can control in their baby: what goes in their gullet.

That being said, I should point out that formula roulette could actually do the trick for your baby or you. Studies looking at colic and other disorders of desperation show that parents happen to be very suggestible. When products and interventions are tested in these studies, the placebo group (the baby getting the inactive drops or product) often shows a remarkable improvement. The idea that things *might* get better has a powerful effect on the exhausted parent.

So switching formulas when your baby is not milk allergic is kind of like believing in Santa Claus. If you don't really believe, there's no chance that your baby will get any better.

YOU SHOULDN'T NEED TO CHANGE FORMULA OVER TASTE

While babies can discriminate between formulas, this remarkable ability should have little impact on what you feed or how you feed your baby. And though soy formula tastes different from cow's milk-based formula, there should be very little difference in the taste across brands. But as we'll see in Chapter 10, your baby may draw the line when it comes to the roadkill flavor of hypoallergenic formulas.

If you feel the need to make a formula change because your baby doesn't seem to like the taste of regular formula, it's harmless to try another formula in the same class—but don't expect much. If your change produces bitter beer face, consult your physician before playing musical formulas. There may be other important reasons why your baby is refusing feeds.

OTHER BABY MILK VARIANTS THAT MIGHT THROW YOU OFF

While I like to see the world as made up of two types of formula, standard and hypoallergenic, there are others. Let me give you the skinny on some of the other milks that you may encounter when you stand in front of the Great Wall of Formula.

SOY FORMULAS

Soy formula was one of the first protein sources used to feed babies back in the dark ages of infant formula. There's nothing wrong with it. In fact, soy formula makes up about 13 percent of all formula consumed by babies. Soy is actually a great protein source for babies, but there are very few reasons why any baby would ever need it. Strictly vegan families go for it since it doesn't contain any kind of animal product. It's also lactose-free, but this is probably irrelevant unless your baby is recovering from a bad tummy virus.

The occasional fussy baby may feel better with soy formula because up to half of babies allergic to milk protein will improve with soy (the other half will react to soy). So while you might get lucky with your allergic baby, I don't recommend soy formula in known or suspected allergic tummy disease.

Soy has had a bad rap of late. There were concerns at one point that the plant hormones found in soy products could cross over to developing children and affect their sexual development. As it turns out, there's no connection between the use of soy infant formulas and hormone derangement in babies and beyond. So if you feel that you must use soy, you can do it with a clear conscience.

LACTOSE-FREE FORMULAS

Lactose intolerance is a nonissue in babies since they're born with all the lactase (lactose-digesting enzyme) they need to digest lactose. This is why breast milk has lactose. And as you'll learn in Chapter 10, removing lactose does nothing to treat milk protein allergy. So while you'll find lactose-free formulas on the market, they serve no purpose in feeding babies—except maybe after a bad tummy virus, if the gut has been injured. Lactose-free formula does more to improve the bottom line of formula manufacturers than it does to improve the digestive state of babies. Lactose is in fact the carbohydrate of choice for young infants, and carbs are the primary source of fuel for your baby. When babies get older, they get their carbohydrates from grains, fruits, and veggies, but as infants they get it from the lactose in breast milk or basic cow's milk formula.

PREEMIE FORMULAS

Premature babies who haven't hit the fourth trimester have different needs from the average baby. While we would like to think that a preemie's nutritional shortcomings are all caught up by the time they leave the hospital nursery, they still have catching up to do after reaching their due date. They need more protein, calcium, and phosphorus compared to their more mature nursery mates. Preemie formulas fill this niche and the needs of the growing preemie. They also contain more fat in the form of *medium-chain triglycerides*, a fat that's more easily absorbed by babies.

A preemie formula is something that your baby starts in the neonatal ICU on the recommendation of your neonatologist. Usually these formulas are continued through the middle of a baby's first year, since the mineral needs for growing former preemies are really unique. Look to your pediatrician for more details.

FOLLOW-UP FORMULAS

If you spend a lot of time in front of the Great Wall of Formula, you'll see that some products take babies through the second half of their first year and into toddlerhood, offering a little more protein and iron for a toddler's growing needs. These formulas haven't had a warm reception among pediatricians and consumers in the United States, because many feel that toddlers can make it just fine with table food and cow's milk. Follow-up formulas, as they are sometimes called, make sense for the superpicky toddler since they offer a more balanced panel of nutrients than milk out of the carton. Otherwise, they represent another way for formula manufacturers to tap into junior's college fund; toddlers do a better job of meeting their nutritional needs than we think.

FORMULA WITH PROBIOTICS AND PREBIOTICS

A great example of how infant formula has grown ever closer to breast milk is the presence of probiotics in today's formulas. Probiotics, as we'll learn in the chapters ahead, are bacteria that have a positive effect on our (or our baby's) health. And as we already know, breast milk is loaded with bugs that play a key role in the creation of a healthy babybiome. These probiotics now found in formula include power bugs like *bifidobacteria* and *L. reuteri*, organisms normally found in breast milk. This gives babies who can't breast-feed a chance at populating their gut with all the right bacteria—along with a chance for all the beneficial health effects that come with it.

Beyond bacteria, some formula manufacturers also add *prebiotics,* which fuel the growth and sustainability of a healthy baby-biome.

CAN I BUY SUPERSTORE OR PHARMACY LABEL FORMULA?

You can absolutely buy superstore or pharmacy label formula, and you can save yourself a bundle by doing so. Infant formulas, whether they are from big brands or off-label superstore varieties, are tightly regulated by the FDA. While there are slightly discernible differences between brands, infant formulas are generally alike with respect to their basic nutritional properties.

DON'T EVEN THINK ABOUT MAKING YOUR OWN FORMULA

On the short list of bad baby-rearing ideas is home brew baby formula. You don't have to look far in Google to find concoctions masquerading as appropriate alternatives to breast milk. Beyond the impurities that your baby is likely to encounter is the risk for infectious contamination, dangerous mineral imbalances, and high likelihood of nutrient shortfalls. Do everything humanly possible to give your baby human milk. And if all else fails, offer the safest and next best option: infant formula.

MORE ON MILK AND HOW IT GETS IN THE TUMMY

THE MILK YOU feed your baby is important, but the way the milk gets into your baby also deserves a little attention.

RISE OF THE MILK GAZERS

Just like parents love to observe, measure, and graph their baby's poo, so it goes for their baby's feeding. Parents are quants and they want to know that what's going in is enough for their baby.

This is a good thing, as this kind of maternal obsession keeps babies nourished and safe. But there's a lot of variation in what babies suck. And, in general, babies are pretty resourceful in terms of making their needs heard.

HOW OFTEN DO BABIES FEED?

Perhaps it's obvious, but how often babies feed depends on how old they are and how hungry they are.

But let's be more specific.

Newborn babies feed about every two or two and a half hours (measured from the start of one feed to the start of the next). Babies should be fed when they're hungry and not by a rigid schedule.

By one month of age you might expect your baby to feed about every three or four hours and one or two times overnight. Expect your breast-fed baby to take approximately eight feeds a day with a couple of snacks.

By three months of age your baby will start to consolidate feeds, so she may take only six or seven feeds per day. At night she may be down to one nighttime feed or, if things are going your way, none at all.

Of course, your mileage may vary. I could go on for pages and pages, but you get the gist.

WHY DOES A ONE-MONTH-OLD BABY FEED EVERY THREE OR FOUR HOURS?

This may seem like a silly question, but I think it's worth a mention. How and why babies feed on the schedules they do is based on *how much they are fed* and *what babies' bodies do with it.*

And as it turns out, the timing is pretty specific.

As we've seen, your baby's stomach starts tiny and ramps up in size as milk production kicks in and metabolic demand picks up. The four to five ounces (or thereabout) that your five-week-old takes at a given feed hits the stomach and fills it up. Since the stomach can only fit about six ounces at that time, your baby declares she's full by slowing down the pace of her feed and stopping (more on your baby's ability to manage her intake in the coming pages).

Over the course of the next 90 to 120 minutes, the stomach slowly releases the milk into the small intestine and digestive hormones and enzymes go to work. As the stomach gets progressively smaller and more empty at two to three hours after her feed, your baby begins to sense the collapse. There is a change in a bunch of hormonal and digestive triggers that feed back to her brain, telling her that the cycle is near complete and it's time to look for more fuel.

As growth spurts happen during the first year, hunger will drive the greedy sucking of higher volumes of milk, which will stretch the stomach further, take it longer to empty, and push the feeding interval longer.

EARLY GROWTH BY THE NUMBERS

During the first four months of life you can expect your baby to gain about an ounce a day or approximately one and a half to two pounds per month. Most healthy infants double their birth weight by four to five months of age and triple it by twelve months. Your baby will grow about ten inches during her first year and another four to five inches during her second year.

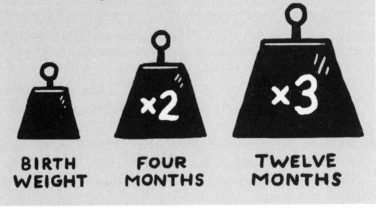

BIRTH WEIGHT　　**FOUR MONTHS**　　**TWELVE MONTHS**

THE SPEED OF THE FEED | A HIDDEN KEY TO BABY WELLNESS

How long it takes your baby to feed is worth mentioning because feeding efficiency is a great indicator of baby wellness. While a baby might be getting what she needs, it's helpful to know *how long it's taking.*

The speed of the feed can vary tremendously from baby to baby, but in general, a formula-fed newborn should be able to finish two and a half ounces within about twenty minutes. If your baby is going through a growth spurt, she might be able to take three or four ounces inside of seven to ten minutes.

Babies who are prone to falling asleep at the breast or bottle may take longer to feed only because they like to doze.

If your baby takes longer than twenty-five minutes to finish her bottle (not including power naps), talk to your pediatrician. While the issue may be as simple as the wrong nipple choice, there are a few small problems that should be checked off the list. These may include things like tongue-tie (a condition that restricts the tongue's range of motion) and acid reflux.

YOUR BABY CAN'T TALK BUT SHE CAN TELL YOU WHEN SHE'S FULL

So how do you know when your baby's full? I'm going to go out on a limb and guess that this is the number one feeding question for new parents. And it's a good question since it isn't always obvious, especially when you've never been responsible for caring for a really small person.

Knowing when your baby is full is all about reading your baby's cues and patterns. On a certain level this can only happen after you know how your baby operates as an individual. Broad, categorical signs aren't as reliable since every baby is different.

In general, babies will tell you they've had enough by slowing down the pace of feeding, pulling away, or dozing off. For the newborn feeding by bottle, this will happen at around two ounces. For the breast-fed infant, look for this to happen after ten minutes or so on each side (keep in mind that things may be touch and go during the first week of breastfeeding while your milk is coming in and your baby is figuring out how to get it).

As a good rule of thumb, a baby should be getting about two and a half ounces of milk per pound of body weight every day. Remember that what a baby takes can vary from day to day and week to week as her metabolic demand changes. Either way, your baby should be getting enough to generate six to eight wet diapers per day. Pee is one of the best indicators that your baby is getting enough to eat.

JUST BECAUSE THE BOTTLE HOLDS FOUR OUNCES DOESN'T MEAN THAT'S ALL SHE NEEDS

Young babies are often fed formula or expressed breast milk (removed with a breast pump) in four-ounce bottles. This works well because the feeding volume of a young baby is typically under four ounces and less milk is wasted. The problem comes at a month or two of age, when your baby's nutritional needs evolve and she likely needs more than four ounces at a sitting. I've seen a bunch of babies fall off their healthy growth curves because their parents inadvertently capped their milk at four ounces and never thought to go any further.

If your baby is goin' and blowin' at the tail end of her little starter bottle, it may be time to try a six-to eight-ounce bottle.

THE FEEDING VOLUME TABLE THAT I DIDN'T WANT TO PUT IN THE BOOK

To fuel your obsessive thinking about whether your baby is getting enough milk, I've included this handy table for you to reference. It offers a very general, ball-park kind of idea of what a baby should be doing. Personally, I don't like these kinds of tables, but I know that if I didn't include one, you'd probably just Google it and then wind up getting your feeding advice from a guy in Singapore trying to sell you herbs.

Remember that your baby is her own little person, and her activity, mood, and more will determine what she wants to take and when.

First days: 10–14 ounces/day (about 2 ounces every three to four hours)
1 month: 18–22 ounces/day (about 4 ounces every four hours)
2 months: 22–28 ounces/day (about 4 ounces 6–7 times per day)
3 months: 25–35 ounces/day (about 4–6 ounces 6 times per day)
6 months: 30–35 ounces/day (about 6–8 ounces 5 times per day)

OVERFEEDING IS OVERRATED

If you've been paying attention to the basics of feeding your baby as discussed thus far, overfeeding isn't anything you should need to worry about. As we'll learn when we talk about the stuff that comes out of babies in Chapter 6, reflux and spit-up is a digestive problem, not a parenting problem. Overfeeding is too often overstated and blamed on poor parental feeding practices.

If you pay attention to your baby's cues, overfeeding is unlikely to be an issue.

HOW LONG IS FORMULA GOOD ONCE YOU'VE MADE IT?
Opened or prepared formula is good for up to forty-eight hours in the fridge. At room temperature, formula should be used within two to four hours. While

you may get away with pushing the limits, remember that formula can begin to harbor harmful bacteria when left open too long.

When in doubt, dump it out.

SLEEPING (OR FUELING) THROUGH THE NIGHT

When it comes to what goes into your baby, the hours when the milk needs to go in can be a point of concern. Especially if those are the wee hours of the morning.

The amount of time that babies go between feedings depends upon (1) how much fuel they need and (2) the capacity of their tummies. The smaller stomachs of newborns can only hold enough to keep them happy for a couple of hours, while two-month-olds can easily hold on to enough milk to satisfy them for four hours or so. Sleepy newborns, however, may need to be awoken to be reminded to feed during the first three or four weeks. This is especially important for the breast-feeding mother who is dependent upon the stimulation of frequent feeding to support her supply.

You may notice that your baby will start to drop her middle-of-the-night feed beginning around two months of age. It's not necessary in this case to arouse her to feed. In fact, this may represent the early beginnings of sleeping through the night.

CEREAL IN THE FORMULA

Every parent wants to game the system when it comes to making their baby sleep at night. And the biggest buzz in parenting groups comes from adding a little cereal to the bottle. It makes some sense: fill 'em up and they'll keep quiet.

In reality, however, this typically doesn't bear out as a sustainable solution.

The addition of cereal to an infant's nighttime bottle is unlikely to stretch out the interval between feeds and it probably won't make any significant difference in the amount of sleep you get. Despite the folksy feeling that cereal will "stick to their ribs," it does little to impact the way the infant tummy pushes, squeezes, and empties—key factors in determining whether your little bundle of milk consumption will wake you up. To add a little hard evidence to the mix, researchers in the *American Journal of Diseases of Children* studied two groups of children, one receiving cereal-supplemented formula and the other getting plain formula. When it came down to sleeping through the night, there was no difference between the two groups.

And a pediatric gastroenterologist's opinion: although it's unlikely to harm your baby, be aware that you may be faced with a constipated baby . . . who won't sleep at night.

More important, we're really not sure how the premature introduction of calories impacts lifelong health and metabolism, which adds another strike against the cereal-in-the-bottle trick.

FEEDING IS NOT ABOUT CONTROL

A lot of modern parenting is about control. Like stool-gazing, we believe that when we measure and graph, we're in control. In modern business there's a saying that you can't manage what you can't measure, and many parents seem to apply that to their babies.

The problem is that babies aren't projects and they have little regard for checklists, timelines, and a predictable flow. Fueling the gut and nurturing a brain is not a process to be micromanaged. Obsessive measuring won't change what they do.

Babies are unpredictable and dynamic. Their needs evolve by the day and the week. This is the process of human development. If you can't bend and move with these changes, you'll be in for a painful ride—or the pushback on your baby's biology will create real problems. And when it comes to feeding, structure can be a problem. The first days of breast-feeding require near constant attention to your baby as a means of establishing a good supply of milk.

Don't get me wrong, structure and order have their place, especially as children get older and more clever.

Of course, we want to know if our babies aren't measuring up. But stress and the pressure to meet metrics is something that can screw up a great feeding relationship. While your baby will ultimately develop her own pattern and rhythm, it's not something that you create.

Once it's clear that a baby is doing what she's supposed to do, pull back, relax, and enjoy.

UNDERSTANDING A BABY'S DIGESTIVE STATE OF WELLNESS

So how do you know if your baby's in a digestive state of wellness? How do you know when she's getting enough or that her gut is doing what it's supposed to do?

Bottom line: *When stuff's coming out, it's a good indicator that there's enough going in.*

More specifically:

Pee. Perhaps the single best indicator that a baby is receiving enough milk is wet diapers. A baby should produce six to eight wet diapers in a twenty-four-hour period. The urine should be light colored and it shouldn't smell very strong. Wet diapers tell us that a baby's fluid intake is up to par. And when milk intake is adequate to meet fluid needs, a baby's nearly always getting what she needs nutritionally.

You can probably stop there, but you can look at a few other things as well.

Other signs of hydration. A baby should have moist lips and even the ability to make little raspberry bubbles around the corner of her mouth. Tears are a great indicator of hydration, but don't look for them until six to twelve weeks of age.

Poo. While a less reliable indicator than pee, your baby will initially poo a handful of times each day. After a month or two of age, this will slow down to once a day or even less. Chapters 8 and 9 will cover the roller coaster of poo frequency and appearance in more detail.

Growth. The ultimate measure of whether a baby's gut is doing what it's supposed to do is how she grows. If she's getting the groceries, she'll build muscle and fat. The most reliable way to know if she's growing is to plot her on a growth curve. This requires weighing her on a consistent scale so that growth can be followed over time in comparison to other babies her age.

WEIGHING BABY (DON'T TRY THIS AT HOME)
I discourage parents from following their baby's weight at home. Why?

- **Reliable info calls for reliable measurement.** Most consumer-grade scales aren't up to par for measuring the subtle differences in growth in a baby.

- **It's hard to know when to get concerned.** Assessing the normal variants of growth takes a lot of experience. Almost universally, self-assessment of growth leads to unnecessary worry.
- **There's no way to act on it.** When there's something to be concerned about, there's no way for you to act on it. You can't control how your baby feeds, and if your baby isn't getting enough, you will likely need the professional help of a pediatrician or lactation consultant to take the right action.

So please don't try this at home. It will just make you crazy. (The only exception is when you're under the care of a lactation consultant. Pre- and postfeeding weights are often used to see if a baby's getting enough.)

MILK: WARM, COLD, OR SOMEWHERE IN BETWEEN

On our growing list of parental preoccupations with feeding is warm milk. We've all been brainwashed into believing that a baby can only drink milk that's been carefully warmed by her mama or papa. While warm milk is fine, your baby is also fine drinking milk at refrigerator or room temperature. There is no evidence that normal variations in temperature impact a baby's sense of fullness or digestion.

But this is a good case where parental impulse tends to trump the evidence. If a parent always wants to give warm milk, that's okay. Just avoid the microwave and warm the milk by immersing the bottle in a basin of warm water.

MILK AND MICROWAVES

While considered a godsend to the modern parent, the microwave can carry hidden dangers when used as a milk warming appliance. Any liquid warmed in a microwave is subject to a phenomenon called onion skinning, where layers of the liquid can heat up to dangerous temperatures. This can lead to superficial burns of your baby's mouth and swallowing tube that can impact normal feeding for days. If you want to serve warm milk, think ahead and place the bottle in a warm bowl of water. Otherwise, milk may be a food better served cold.

FOUR THINGS TO KNOW ABOUT WATER AND YOUR BABY

Surely a baby doesn't live on milk alone, you're thinking. Actually, they do. But since your baby is 78 percent water, there are a few things to remember about water and when we put it into a baby.

1. YOUR BABY DOESN'T NEED EXTRA WATER

During the first six months, your baby gets enough fluid from breast milk or formula. Healthy infants usually require no supplemental water except when exposed to unusually hot weather. Even in this situation, supplemental water should not exceed four ounces per day in children under six months. Once a child reaches six months and is eating solids, her need for fluid other than breast milk or formula will increase. Between six and twelve months, a baby's supplemental fluid intake should probably be limited to ten ounces a day.

2. WATER OCCUPIES CRITICAL GUT REAL ESTATE FOR THE GROWING BABY

When your baby's stomach is full of water she'll have no room for the fat, protein, and calories needed for growth. While this may be a good strategy for mamas looking to lose their baby weight, it's not so good for a growing baby.

3. DON'T WORRY ABOUT FLUORIDE UNTIL AFTER SIX MONTHS

There's no need to supplement your breast- or formula-fed baby with fluoride before six months of age. More specifically, be sure not to prepare your powder or concentrate formula with fluoridated water since it can lead to fluorosis, a condition where the teeth have a funny discoloration from excess fluoride supplementation. Bottled water low in fluoride is often labeled as deionized, demineralized, or distilled. Low fluoride water specially sold for "nursery use" is typically considered safe with respect to fluoride. And the FDA mandates that products that contain supplemental fluoride be labeled as such, so be sure to check the labels.

Regarding run-of-the-mill bottled water, fluoride levels can vary depending upon the source and whether it's undergone reverse osmosis or filtering. Most run on the low end, but it's worth checking the fluoride level of your brand if you choose the option of using bottled water.

After the first six months, the need for fluoride supplementation depends on the fluoride concentration of the water in your community or the water your baby drinks.

Be sure to get a firm recommendation from your local pediatrician.

4. DON'T DRINK THE WATER

The water used to prepare infant formula should be boiled for the infant less than three months of age. Outbreaks of infectious diarrhea related to contaminated municipal water supplies are occasionally reported in the United States, but the risk is minimal and doesn't warrant sterilization for the older infant and child.

(If you've been paying attention, Looking Out for Number Two *has been pushing the idea that bacteria are good for your baby. Remember that we're talking about the right bacteria at the right time. We still need to do everything possible to keep our babies from pathogens. Those are bacteria that cause disease.)*

To sterilize water, bring it to a boil for one minute, but no longer. Prolonged boiling can cause minerals and impurities naturally found in the water to become concentrated to levels dangerous for baby.

Bottled water from a trusted source is a solid option.

Baby Food and Other Forms of Advanced Bowel Fuel

M ILK IS BIG, BUT THERE'S NOTHING BIGGER THAN TAKING YOUR BABY to the next great step in bowel fuel: solid food. While milk was all about breast or bottle, the world of solid food brings your baby closer to eating like a real person. But starting solids comes with a new set of issues.

THE CONVERSATION OF FEEDING

WE'RE RAISING A GENERATION OF HELICOPTER FEEDERS

I may be a super-duper subspecialist who spends his days working with digestive and nutritional problems in the largest children's hospital in America, but even I think we've gone too far in shaping feeding around the idea of rocket-science nutrients. We've taken the feeding relationship between a mother and baby and made it into some kind of evidence-based scientific encounter. We've created a generation of **helicopter feeders**.

As helicopter feeders, we fuel our babies according to rules and regulations, with the belief that if we deviate, our kids will die.

Instead, we should focus on a healthy balance of fresh foods. When we stick to cultivating a palate for a variety of real foods with a natural array of colors and shapes, the numbers and the nutrients take care of themselves. In fact, when delivered in their unprocessed state, nutrients are able to work together in ways that we're just beginning to understand. While your options for whole foods may be limited during the first months of life, it shouldn't stop you from helping to build in variety.

While we've advanced the science of understanding our food, the process of getting that food into your baby is a maternal/paternal art that needs little in the way of medical or scientific regulation.

FEEDING A BABY IS LIKE A CONVERSATION

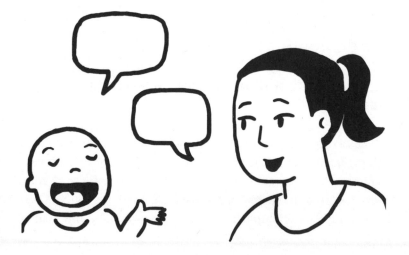

When it comes to feeding, rules are tricky because every baby and every parent is different. Each will offer and take food in a way that's unique. So every feeding encounter between a parent and a baby is something of a conversation. And when we think about good conversation, most of us would agree that both parties have to listen to each other before they can respond in a meaningful way. Successful feeding is no different and requires that you listen to your baby and follow her lead. Only you can know and understand the rhythm of your baby's patterns. This failure to really understand your baby's signals is one of the fundamental problems behind so many feeding difficulties that new parents encounter.

Listen to your baby and recognize that this conversation should be inspiring, not stressful.

As parents starting kids on solids, we're preoccupied with gagging and choking, "reactions," and the fear that our baby may not be getting enough. But the truth of the matter is that actual choking in babies is a rarity, reactions to food are less common than you think, and babies do an amazing job of taking in what they need. Instead, what we should be concerned with is setting the stage for a healthy lifelong relationship with food. That's the most important nutritional legacy you can leave for your kids, and it begins by letting go of the stuff that's not worth worrying about, which I will point out in the coming sections.

So let's move beyond milk to the realities and myths of solid food and other things used to fuel your baby.

WHEN TO PUT IN FOOD | THE NOT-SO-MYSTERIOUS REALITY OF FEEDING

THE CRAZY RACE TO START SOLIDS

I don't think there's a bigger question in the first year of life than when to start solid food. In fact, there's a huge sense of urgency among some families. The American Academy of Pediatrics recommends exclusive breast-feeding (that's just breast milk without food) for six months. Remember that there's only so much real estate in the stomach. When your baby starts solids, she begins the slow slide away from milk toward regular food. Holding solids until six months optimizes a baby's exposure to breast milk and increases the odds that she'll breast-feed longer.

If you cheat the system, you're definitely not alone. Data from the Centers for Disease Control and the FDA suggest that by four months of age 40 percent of infants have consumed cereal and 17 percent have had fruits and veggies. But if you're gunning to be part of this stat, you may want to think through why.

Your baby will get most of what she needs from breast milk or formula until at least halfway through her first year. Babies don't sleep better with solids and there's certainly no evidence that it makes them happier. Instead, forcing food on your baby before four months of age is associated with higher rates of weight gain and the potential for later obesity.

Sure, the photo ops will come earlier, but those can wait. Beyond keeping up with someone else's expectation of what you should or could be doing, there's no logic behind pushing food early.

THE ALMOST-ADULT GUT IN YOUR BABY'S BODY

We talk about babies' readiness to feed but rarely discuss their gut's readiness for food. As it turns out, a baby's intestinal tract is primed and ready to take on all nutrients by two to three months of age. In effect, there's nothing babies can't absorb or digest by the time they reach six months, the age of starting solids. We're not advocating for schnitzel and fettuccine at this point, just illustrating that digestive maturity makes solids of most types possible by four to six months of age. And remember that beyond what the gut can process, food needs to get to the lips, over the tongue, and down the pipe. This takes a mature chewing and swallowing apparatus, which takes months to get into shape. So first things first.

THE MINIMUM MECHANICS FOR EATING

Another reason for lying back a bit when it comes to starting solids is to be sure that your baby's in shape to take the food plunge.

Here are a few things your baby needs to be able to do before you offer the spoon:

- **Maintain head and trunk stability.** Your baby needs to be able to sit with little support and hold her head up. This makes sense—just try eating with your chin on your chest.
- **Show mature mouth mechanics.** Just as the baby body goes through stages of development like standing and walking, the mouth has its own not-so-obvious stages. Your baby needs the ability to open her mouth and make up and down and rotary movements of the jaw.
- **Demonstrate the ability to just say no. Kind of.** Although six-month-olds can't say no, they have ways of getting their point across. Head stability and the ability to open and close their mouth is important, because they have to be able to turn away and tell you when they're not into barley and peas. The ability to open their mouth and lean forward

can send another message about what they want and how quickly.

- **Showcase tongue talent.** The extrusion reflex that exists early in life to keep solids out of the mouth gives way to a tongue that can take food, push it to the side, and, ultimately, push it to the back of the mouth. This one's hard to see from across the room, but you'll know what I mean when you start feeding.
- **Stares longingly as food goes into your mouth.** Or better, your baby reaches as the food goes from your plate to your mouth. This doesn't need a lot of explanation. Suffice it to say that babies are smarter than you think when it comes to food.

Typically, these baby body skills kick in at around four to seven months of age, but your mileage may vary. And again, holding food until six months takes the stress of testing feeding readiness out of the equation.

Even if your child isn't quite there yet, you can always bring her to the table with you. Having your child at the table introduces her to the social aspect of feeding.

THE FEEDING POLICE

As a parent there's no shortage of entitled, self-appointed know-it-alls willing to impose their child-rearing and health standards on you. This is never more evident than when it comes to feeding and nutrition. These sanctimonious guilt-trippers materialize when you're pregnant and will find you as long as you have kids. I call them the feeding police.

The feeding police patrol playgroups, playgrounds, pediatrician waiting rooms, Facebook feeds, and any place frequented by young, impressionable parents. They offer advice when it's not solicited and hold hard-edged opinions on just about everything. Most important, deviance from their self-imposed standard of how, when, and what to do with a child typically comes with the veiled threat that something really bad might happen to your baby. Mandated milk warming is just one example of a common point for meddling nutritional do-gooders. As we've seen, there's no evidence that warm versus room temperature versus cool will impact your baby's capacity for a bright future—and yet the feeding police continue to insist that milk should only be delivered warm.

Peer support is a critical part of parenting. Choose your friends wisely, be careful who you listen to, and remember that you know more than you think you do.

THE TIMELESS MYSTERY OF STARTING SOLIDS IN THE GROWING PREEMIE

Feeding a former premature baby is a challenge because there's a tension between a baby's actual age and their corrected age with regard to things like starting solids. What age do you use and what do you do? When it comes to the decision to start solids, use a growing preemie's corrected age and then look to see if they meet the minimum mechanics for feeding. Developmental readiness more than age should be considered as the most important factor when deciding when to pull the trigger (or spoon) with your ex-preemie.

You'll probably find your baby's ready point falls somewhere between their actual and corrected age. When in doubt, err on the side of waiting.

THE IMPORTANCE OF SOLIDS AND HOW LONG YOU CAN WAIT

Okay, we said that there's no rush to start solids (and for the record, "solids" are anything that normally doesn't come out of a bottle or boob—that includes squishy pureed foods). But let's look at the flip side of feeding and bring up the question asked far less often: How long can a baby wait for solids? The discussion brings up some key elements of solid feeding and why pediatricians recommend what we do.

NUTRIENTS AND OTHER SMALL THINGS

Although most babies will do fine with milk alone through six months, some nutrients and minerals, like iron and zinc, make solids a practical necessity after that point. So, for the nutrients alone, waiting much beyond seven months isn't a great idea. You can, however, work around this with professional input.

SENSATION AND THE TOLERANCE OF TEXTURE

Perhaps a bigger issue with starting solids is the experience of understanding and knowing what to do with it. In fact, early feeding is more a sensory experience than a nutritional exchange. Between seven months and a year, babies enter a critical period where they learn to handle lumps and bumps in their food. Eating pureed food is for amateurs. But knowing how to handle lumps mixed in with puree, crunchy food, or even the dense texture of meat takes experience and practice.

Late in the first year your baby will learn how to deal with these different sensory experiences. This will be invisible to you unless your baby has not experienced varying textures by her first birthday. Not seeing some of these funky textures during that developmental window can later lead to a kind of panic attack with gagging and anxiety. As a child is repeatedly exposed to a sensation that she doesn't know how to handle, and as the anxiety response gets reinforced, it can create a condition called an **oral aversion**.

More on this later, but exposing a baby to food during this key window of sensory opportunity represents a crucial element in feeding development. And it's a good reason to not wait too long.

WHAT TO FEED YOUR BABY

In the big picture of raising your baby, early feeding is all about the sequential transition from liquid to solid stuff. After six months of milk, your baby will start with near liquid consistency mush and progressively advance to things that she can actually chew around her first birthday. There's a lot going on during this transition, and the whole sequence is centered on getting your baby comfortable with the progression. Each step is a new sensation and calls for new oral skills. Each step also depends on the one before it.

So we've got a baby, mouth open, leaning forward and ready. Let's talk about how to get things going.

GETTING STARTED

START 'EM ONCE A DAY WHEN THEIR BRAINS—AND BELLIES— ARE WIDE OPEN

Start with one feed a day to get things going. You can feed twice, but your baby will have enough on her plate (or in that itty-bitty colorful bowl) with just one.

- **Leverage the rise-and-shine mind-set.** You can feed your baby at any time of day, but I recommend the morning, when the baby mind is fresh and open to the potential new experience of mushy cereal and veggies. Remember that food is a radical sensory experience for a baby. If she's pooped or overstimulated, the concentration, focus, and receptiveness necessary to form a little ball of ready-to-swallow food (often referred to as a "bolus" by feeding professionals) and casually shoot it to the back of the mouth just won't happen.
- **Spoon-feed with a bottle chaser.** Deliver that first feed on an empty stomach. Your odds of digestive success are slim if she's just polished off a six-ounce bottle.

START SMALL AND MIX TO PERFECTION

Your baby is effectively a pro with liquid by six months. So the best natural segue into solids is to create a blend that's not too threatening. If you're using cereal, start with one tablespoon of boxed cereal flakes and mix it in a bowl with breast milk or formula to reach a slurry consistency. When it pours off the spoon easily, you're there.

SET THE MOOD AND THE SPACE

Consistency is superhelpful in mealtime routines. Starting early with solid routines will set the pace and rhythm of what you do, or more important, what your baby does with food. This begins with a consistent space and place for feeding.

- **Baby should remain seated in the full-upright position.** Be sure your baby is positioned as close to a full-upright position as possible. While you may never have eaten oatmeal in a semireclined position on the sofa, you can probably appreciate that it may not go well.
- **Be consistent with where you feed.** When you feed with the same bowl in the same high chair positioned in a fixed space, your baby will begin to associate all the crazy goodness of feeding with landing square in that chair. In fact, a whole bunch of physiologic things will start to trigger into motion once your child understands that it's feeding time (gut hormones, salivation, digestive juices, etc.).
- **Be connected and practice eye contact.** The initiation of feeding is not a time for multitasking (for you or your baby). Eating solids requires real baby concentration, so limit distractions.
- **Bring your potentially annoying good morning face.** The attitude you show up with will go a long way in shaping how receptive your child will be to that first feed or the new, strange-tasting stuff that shows up four months later. How you look and how you behave around feeding or when delivering that bite will impact how she sees her food and the experience of feeding.

Attitude, like so many other things with your kids, will take you far.

DON'T FEAR THE EXTRUSION AND OTHER PESKY REFLEXES

With that first spoonful you'll find the initial reaction is a crazy pop-out move with the tongue. You put it in and out it comes. You put it back in and it comes out again.

This natural reaction to "tongue" out anything that feels funny is referred to as the *extrusion reflex*. This short-lived and slightly annoying protective reflex should be handled with gentle persistence. Continue to offer a daily feed consisting of four or five spoonfuls (or attempted spoonfuls). Understand that during the first week of starting food, most of that food will wind up someplace other than her stomach.

You'll read in lesser parenting manuals that a sign of feeding readiness is the ability to keep food in the mouth. If we followed advice like this, all of us would still be exclusively breast-feeding. Even for a baby who's ready, extrusion rejection is part of healthy feeding development and it's something every baby needs to get over.

Accept it. Roll with it. Take pictures of it. Just make sure you have a fresh supply of bibs.

A WORD ABOUT SCHEDULES, STRUCTURE, AND FEEDING

Forget everything I told you until now about schedules. From this moment forward, you want to think about fashioning a basic schedule for your baby.

Back during the early weeks of life, when you were just starting out with breast- or bottle-feeding, schedules had the potential to corrupt what nature is designed to do: create a natural pattern and rhythm of healthy milk production and consumption. Early on, schedules are bad for babies.

At this point, though, beginning to understand the social process and structure of feeding is critical to the development of both a healthy digestive system and good eating habits. From here on out, structure is a good thing when it comes to a child's eating and sleeping.

IS THERE A CRITICAL ORDER OF INTRODUCTION OF FOOD?

Nothing about feeding is critical.

In fact, the only real constant when it comes to starting solids is the recommendation that you kick things off with cereal. The reason for this is that babies tend to be short on iron later in their first year, and cereal is a rich source of iron.

Here are a few other thoughts on sequencing solids.

CHOOSE OATMEAL OVER RICE CEREAL TO AVOID CONSTIPATION

A recent study showed that oatmeal is less constipating in babies and carries with it all the glorious iron found in rice. So if hard, painful, bottom-tearing turds are your baby's problem, give oatmeal a whirl. Or just avoid any potential problems by using oatmeal from the start.

BEYOND CEREAL, PROCEED WITH WHATEVER FOOD YOU LIKE

The only consideration to keep in mind is that foods should be introduced one at a time in order to identify any type of intolerance or allergy (more on this in Chapter 10). You can introduce new foods around four days after a previous food has been introduced, as reactions in the gut sometimes need a few days to become apparent.

STARTING SOLIDS WITH MEAT (AND OTHER CRAZY IDEAS)

Growing concern over iron intake in infancy has prompted some leading nutritionists and pediatricians to advocate the initiation of solids with meat. While your baby's iron intake with cereal should be fine, knowing that some of pediatrics' leading experts have suggested kicking off with meat should support the idea that the order of operations is not critical.

THE MYTH OF VEGGIES BEFORE FRUITS (AND OTHER URBAN FEEDING LEGENDS)

Let's put this famed myth to bed: There's no evidence that the order of introduction of different foods has any influence on the outcome of taste preference. And despite the ever-popular urban legend of veggies before fruit, starting with fruits before veggies won't doom your child to a life of never eating her vegetables. Sequence is a lot less important than you think. If you find yourself deliberating over which comes first, sweet potatoes or green beans, ask yourself one question: Will this matter on the day of her college graduation?

THE ART OF KNOWING WHEN YOUR BABY IS TOPPED OFF

If you don't know how to figure out if your baby's full, you're in good company. I spent six years training in pediatrics and nutrition, and when we brought my son home I had no idea when he was full. As a parent, you'll need to figure out some things in real time, independent of how educated you are. This happens to be one of them. Knowing when your baby has had enough is something of an art. It comes down to understanding your baby and her signals, and it's part of the conversation that I talked about at the beginning of the chapter. But I can still provide some direction.

It's difficult to describe, but when a baby's in the middle of a bowl of squash, you can almost read them by what they're doing. Their posture and expression can tell you what's happening in their stomachs. A hungry baby in the middle of an amazing bowl of pureed peas will typically look for that next bite. You can almost see and feel their anticipation and you may even see them looking into the bowl.

As soon as you begin to see the pace of the feed taper off, that should serve as a cue that you're almost there. A clear sign that they're becoming topped off is when they're more easily distracted by things going on in the kitchen or at the table. At this point you should remark that the next spoonful is the last bite, indicating that feeding time is over.

It's important to set expectations early about the finality of the feeding encounter. Defining firm boundaries now is critical training for the later encounters that you'll have with your temperamental toddler.

STAGING YOUR BABY FOOD

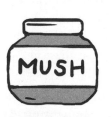 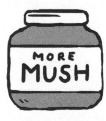 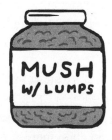

STAGE 1   STAGE 2   STAGE 3

If you choose to feed your baby prepared baby food, you'll need to understand the staging system. So sit down, grab your highlighter, and pay attention.

The staging of baby food by manufacturers is a pretty arbitrary system of grading food by consistency or lumpiness. **Stage one** is effectively liquidlike, pureed food and **stage three** is pureed food with moderately large residual lumps of solid food. **Stage two** is closer in consistency to stage one foods, but it is often sold in larger jars to meet the appetite of growing babies. Beyond the size of the jar, stage two foods tend to be available in a more tantalizing array of varieties (with more than one ingredient) when compared to stage one.

ADVANCING FOOD STAGES DOESN'T REQUIRE A MEDICAL LICENSE

Advancing from puree to something more lumpy requires neither a medical license nor permission from your pediatrician. This is a decision that will come from understanding your baby and her progress.

If your baby is putting away her stage ones and takes a small variety of fruits and vegetables (4–6), take the leap to stage two for variety and convenience. Be aware of the addition of new fruits, veggies, and other ingredients that may not have been present in her individual stage one servings, and keep this in mind in the event of a reaction.

IF YOUR BABY'S SMART, SHE'LL SKIP STAGE THREE

More advanced textured foods (stage three) should be offered around eight months of age. But if your baby is bellying up to the family table and eating with you at least once a day, she may become more interested in your warm, freshly smooshed mashed potatoes than her mysterious "beef dinner." Once babies experience the reality of real food, they'll often never make it to stage three. And that's fine. This is part of the flexibility of feeding that will make the conversation a success.

STAGE YOUR HOMEMADE FOOD TO DELIVER INCREASING TEXTURE

If you choose to prepare your own foods, you will want to progressively advance the texture of your baby's food beginning around eight months of age. Exposure to texture is a critical first step to understanding and advancing to more complex foods.

HOW LONG IS BABY FOOD GOOD FOR ONCE IT'S OPENED?

Once baby food is opened, it can last forty-eight to seventy-two hours, as long as you aren't putting the used spoon back in the jar. If you feed from the jar and use the same spoon to get another portion, you are committing the cardinal sin of "double dipping." If you double dip, don't save the leftover portion. I recommend putting your estimated serving in a bowl before the feed in case she doesn't finish, and then you can save the remainder in the jar.

TEETH ARE OVERRATED

There isn't a single decision you will need to make about feeding during the first year of life that will involve knowing how

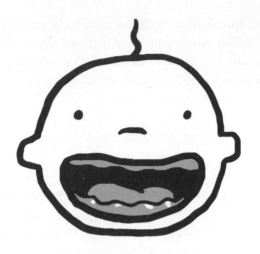

many teeth your baby has. From puree to food with lumps and on to basic table food, all you need to worry about is whether it can be squished between your thumb and index finger.

In fact, all you really need to know is if your baby has gums. If she has gums, you're good to go.

The teeth that do the heavy lifting when it comes to chewing are the molars, and those won't be in play until she's twelve to eighteen months. If you buy the harebrained logic that babies can't advance textures without some kind of magical tooth count, you may find yourself in trouble with a baby who has no idea what to do when food hits her tongue. Don't be that parent.

Advance textures in the way we discussed and make sure that whatever you give can easily be squished.

BABY TASTE PREFERENCE | OR WHY IT MAY TAKE FIFTEEN SHOTS TO SINK ONE

A baby has the ability to discern tastes long before solids are started. And as soon as a baby has the capacity to close her mouth, turn away, pull back, or put on a bitter beer face, she's demonstrating her preference. While most of us would like to believe that we're in control of everything that our babies do, these preferences for taste begin early. In fact, most taste quirks are short-lived and rarely evolve into lifelong patterns. The source of today's sour face could be tomorrow's obsession.

With that said, there's the reality of the fickle infant palate and the question of what actually constitutes rejection. As it turns out, while a baby may not *appear* to like something, what's more likely is that they may not really *know* what they like. **Studies suggest that it may take up to fifteen introductions for a baby to accept a new food.**

So is it critical that you burn through fifteen jars of pureed squash to get your baby hooked? Since no baby lives or dies by pureed squash . . . probably not. The point is that while babies may look fickle, they're simply uncommitted.

And don't let your preferences bias your baby. Just because you don't like spinach or kiwi doesn't mean your baby won't. Your baby is a clean slate. Let her grow to develop her own taste preferences.

SHOULD YOU MAKE YOUR OWN BABY FOOD?

The decision to prepare your own food or offer jarred food is a big one for a lot of parents. Feeding is an emotional event, and for some parents, the knowledge of what they prepare on their own and the hands-on love that's part of their food preparation make homemade baby food a clear option.

As far as what's *nutritious*, that can mean any number of

things depending upon your POV, what you're used to eating, and how you define nutrition. While it can be argued that vacuum-sealed jarred vegetables may have subtle nutritional differences when compared with kitchen prepared vegetables, the differences aren't significant enough to justify turning your kitchen into a near-professional food processing center. Single-ingredient stage one foods from the major manufacturers typically consist of only pureed fruits and vegetables, with nothing else added. More advanced stages of foods may contain artificial colors (names beginning with FD&C, which indicate the FDA has approved the colorant for use in foods, drugs, and cosmetics), sweeteners, sugar, and salt. So watch your labels, as your mileage may vary.

And at the end of the day, it's what works for you.

HOMEMADE FOODS TO AVOID

If you do make your own baby food, you may be told to avoid beets, squash, turnips, carrots, spinach, and collard greens because these vegetables contain compounds called nitrates that can interfere with the way red blood cells transport oxygen around the body. The American Academy of Pediatrics guidelines recommend avoiding these vegetables during the first three months of life (the cells most susceptible to nitrates are the fetal red blood cells, which are typically gone by this age). Since this reaction is rare to begin with—and given that you won't be fueling your baby's gut with solids until after six months—you should have nothing to worry about.

For the record, manufacturers monitor their products for safe levels of nitrates.

BEWARE THE ORGANIC TRAP

The baby food market has crafted a class divide with two types of food: organic and regular. Organic is promoted as premium in all regards; regular has become the second-class citizen or the dirty food. And parents will go broke offering their baby what they perceive to be the best there is.

Studies show that organic baby food is not measurably different from its standard-issue shelf-mates when it comes to pesticides and things that don't belong. But, just to be sure, we buy organic. Thus the trap. Of course we should be careful about how our food is sourced, but the exposure risk at this level is negligible to unmeasurable. And like so many other parts of parenting, we have to choose where to allocate our energy and our cash.

Save the organic splurge for when you're choosing berries, fresh vegetables, and other pesticide-risky foods once your baby is eating them after a year. And remember that "all natural" doesn't mean organic or more healthy. All natural sugar and regular sugar both provide your baby with the same empty calories at the end of the day.

MEAT IS NOT EVIL

Meat can be introduced anytime after six months of age. Babies can survive without meat, but as mentioned previously it's also a terrific source of protein and iron. While meat may be perceived as less healthy by cholesterol-conscious adults, it becomes important when you consider that the intake of iron-rich cereal goes down later in the first year as older babies expand their diets. And not all iron is created equal. The type of iron found in meat is absorbed more efficiently than that found in cereals or fortified foods.

So despite the fact that infants can get by without meat, don't ignore the power and potential that it packs.

GAGGING AS A SWALLOWING SPEED BUMP

No discussion about what goes into a baby could be complete without a discussion of gagging. Parents universally freak out when their babies gag—that's just part of the job description. But it's actually a very natural reaction as your baby learns to eat.

Here's why your baby generates this frightening response to food:

- **Gagging because they don't know what else to do.** All babies gag from time to time. It's what you do when you're nine months old and you don't know what to do with that itty-bitty fiber strand in your overcooked zucchini. It's part of the natural process of learning how to manipulate and swallow foods of different sizes and textures.
- **Gagging to protect the windpipe.** While gagging may look like a life-threatening event, it's actually a sophisticated safeguard designed to keep food from dropping into the windpipe where it really would constitute a life-threatening event. Should food or milk head the wrong direction toward the airway, the muscles of the pharynx intervene and force that food back from where it came. So as hard as it may be, try to think of gagging as your friend. Or your baby's friend.
- **Choking is what gagging is trying to prevent.** If gagging is the protective reflex, choking is what that reflex is trying to prevent. True choking is what happens when food actually gets into the airway and causes a critical blockage of air. The hallmark of the choking child is the silent absence of noise

and airflow. It's unmistakable. Since air can neither move in or out, the child will appear frozen and terrified. As opposed to many of the things that parents get excited about, this truly constitutes an emergency. Fortunately, true choking is a rare event.

Gagging with food should be a rare thing with your baby. If it isn't, your first stop needs to be with your pediatrician, so that he or she can have a look-see.

WHAT TO DO IF YOUR BABY GAGS WHEN YOU ADVANCE TEXTURES

Beyond the occasional event, consistent gagging, especially when advancing textures, can mean your baby has an underlying problem.

One of the most common reasons for regular gagging is what's called a **sensory aversion**. This is a kind of baby panic attack experienced when faced with an unknown mouth situation. Remember that knowing what to do with your mouth and tongue when experiencing lumps and bumps in food takes some practice. If a baby hasn't sorted out what to do with those lumps and bumps by late in the first year, they'll be rejected with a panicky gag.

The baby's impulse here is to get the food out of her mouth because it's weird, foreign, and potentially threatening. And each time we retry the same texture and elicit the same ugly gag, the baby, her brain, and her mouth sensors become experienced. This causes an earlier and more intense reaction with the next spoonful.

If this type of consistent gagging response isn't addressed, your baby will have a hard time handling the texture in question. This is a situation where a baby needs a formal assessment by a speech pathologist or occupational therapist experienced in infant feeding.

Usually a gagging problem improves with therapy, but this can take weeks to months to turn around.

SQUASH AS HAIR GEL | FEEDING IS A MULTISENSORY EXPERIENCE

So a baby's aversion to textures is something best prevented rather than treated. And one of the most important ways to get babies comfortable with different food textures and to prevent aversion is to let them get dirty with their food. Food on the lips, face, hands, and scalp all contribute to the brain growing comfortable with something. Feeding is a multisensory experience, and facilitating that through exposure on the skin is crucial.

Lots of moms like to keep that puss squeaky clean during feeding, fastidiously wiping between spoonfuls to keep things free and clear. But just like with bacteria, an obsession with cleanliness when it comes to baby food can contribute to a baby's issues. Try to embrace the mess, at least until mealtime is over.

STEP AWAY FROM THE HIGH CHAIR AND NOBODY GETS HURT | WHEN TO END THE CONVERSATION

Knowing when *not to feed* a baby is as important as knowing *when to feed*. More specifically, knowing when to put the spoon down is a little like knowing when to de-escalate an argument with your spouse. It's a fine line that requires social sense, maturity, and appreciation of the big picture.

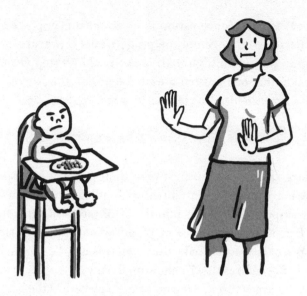

Here's why you should think long and hard before starting a food fight: *fighting creates feeding tension.*

Forcing a baby to do what you want her to do with her mouth and stomach sets a dangerous precedent about food, emotions, and the experience of fueling the body. Nothing about feeding should ever be forced. There are no exceptions to this.

UNDERSTAND THE DIVISION OF RESPONSIBILITY

Feeding therapist Ellyn Satter has described the **Division of Responsibility,** which suggests that when feeding, the responsibilities of the parent are separate and different from those of the child. A parent's job is to prepare and deliver a meal. A child's is to eat it according to what she needs. The two jobs shall never cross. More specifically, it is not a parent's job to make a child eat. We are simply facilitators of fuel for our children.

In my practice, the first step in healing the desperately dysfunctional feeding conversation is to invoke and apply the Division of Responsibility. Simply helping parents to prepare, deliver, and step away from the high chair is a critical first step. Over time, the tension that had created a wedge between the baby and her food dissolves, and feeding takes a more natural course.

BABIES MAY SKIP A MEAL. OR TWO.

As children approach their first year, their patterns of intake and appetite may become less predictable. Toddlers, for example, frequently skip meals. What's important in terms of intake is not what happens during any one meal, but what happens during the course of a baby's week. And while even this may be impossible to measure, the end result will show on a baby's growth curve. Despite what we may think, a normal rate of growth is the best indicator that you're meeting your baby's needs.

Parents make lousy dietitians, and babies have a better sense of what they're doing than we can appreciate.

YOUR BABY WON'T DIE WITHOUT YELLOW VEGETABLES

There's no food that a baby can't live without. If you're hell-bent on the life-or-death acceptance of yellow vegetables, that's your problem, not your baby's. While there may be bad diets, there are no bad foods or critical foods. Every child's palate and diet is a little different. Accept this and you'll likely never need to think about the Division of Responsibility.

You know it's time to end the conversation when feeding becomes more about your issues than about your baby's needs.

DON'T WORRY ABOUT GETTING THE LAST WORD—LEAVE "ONE MORE BITE" AT THE DOOR

Watch a young parent feed a young baby and you'll always see them try to get in the last word. But "one more bite" should play no part in your feeding conversations. Like a kind of nutritional one-upsmanship, this timeless push to get your baby to eat one more spoonful of something is more about you and your fear of malnutrition than it is about what your baby needs.

TABLE FOOD AND BEYOND

TABLE FOOD IS a huge step because it marks the move from baby to small person who fits in with the rest of the family.

WHEN TO START USING TABLE FOOD AS BABY FUEL

So when is it safe to start fueling your baby's gut with table food? It depends on what you're calling table food. To some this is food in the form that we would eat it as adults. To others, table food is anything that doesn't come from a baby food jar. Let's consider table food as stuff that we may eat, but perhaps in a form that's prepared for a baby or toddler.

More simply put, table food is the stuff that comes off our plate.

What makes the table food transition dicey is that there isn't a hard trigger point for table food. The decision to start baby food is a little clearer. But if you pay attention, beginning around eight months of age, most babies begin to take interest in what's out there beyond the high chair. This may be limited to curiosity about the colors and shapes on your plate. Some babies, however, will begin to turn down their baby food as a sign that they're ready for something more advanced. This is a sure sign that they're getting more adventurous.

If your baby's eight months old and you suspect that she's tired of peas and barley, try offering some unseasoned mashed potato or squash from your plate. You'll know pretty quickly if it was the right move.

WHAT WE CAN LEARN FROM GRANDMA

While you may believe that Grandma's full of out-dated parenting beliefs, most grandmothers bring an instinctive "let's go for it" attitude to the high chair. They bring the fifty-thousand-foot view without the inhibitions that hold new parents back, and that helps them push the limits of what babies can do with food.

Sometimes this mind-set can pay off. I recently had an eight-month-old baby who had developed a feeding aversion to the bottle due to acid reflux (that's when they learn to hate to swallow because they think it's going to hurt; reflux is covered in detail in Chapter 6).This baby was really frustrating to feed because it took her so long to finish a bottle. So Grandma thought that it might be interesting to feed this baby with a regular cup (closely supervised, of course). As it turns out, the baby fed better with a cup than she did with a bottle, since it was the sucking of the bottle that she associated with the pain.

While we don't routinely feed eight-month-olds with regular cups, it is a strategy that can be used in this age group when intake with a bottle is problematic. And while we always want to partner with our pediatricians and feeding therapists on creative approaches to feeding, parents need more of this can-do attitude. This is why I love grandparents.

BABIES AND THEIR JUICE

So where does juice fit in between breast milk and table food?

Let's start with an incontrovertible nutrition fact: no baby needs juice. Consider it an extra or an add-on.

But just like we've been trained to think that ketchup is a vegetable, we've been brainwashed to believe that juices serve as a valuable source of vitamins and minerals. In fact, those nutrients come through a well-balanced diet including breast milk, solids, and sometimes ketchup.

While it's safe to offer juice as early as six months of age, a good goal might be to wait until she's drinking from a sippy cup. This may encourage the transition to an alternate, more age-appropriate way of drinking.

Limit juice to four to six ounces a day, and look at it as a way to provide variety and fluid to her diet. I like to cut juice in half with water, since that cuts added sugar by half. I'm also a fan of flavored waters as a nonmilk source of fluid.

WHEN TO START YOGURT AND OTHER MILKLIKE THINGS

Yogurt is a center of many nutrition discussions because its texture makes it well suited for babies, yet it's essentially a milk product. Remember that milk-based foods like yogurt are basically milk in solid form.

The issue with straight cow's milk in babies early in life is that it can be tough on the lining of the intestine. However, small amounts are fine. And as your baby advances to table foods, she'll be exposed increasingly to cow's milk.

I recommend holding yogurt until eight months with daily quantities limited to two to four ounces per day. Stick with the plain, nonsweetened variety and add your own soft, minced fruit to add flavor. Yogurt should be withheld in babies with known milk allergy.

MOVING TO THREE SQUARE MEALS A DAY

Just as soon as a baby is used to the concept of solid food, it's reasonable to transition her to three meals a day just like the rest of the family. A good time to do this is around seven months, though you can do this a bit earlier or later.

The move to three square meals a day is an exciting milestone because it signals that your baby is starting to eat like other members of the family. Assuming that you eat together as a family at least once or twice a day, this emerging social experience of feeding is important because it showcases to a baby what's expected of them.

Truth be told, the idea of three meals a day is a relatively arbitrary pattern of feeding. You may eat two big meals a day or four smaller ones. Our interval of feeding is socially driven and somewhat based on what our stomachs can allow.

But whatever your feeding schedule may be, the structure becomes important late in the first year. Just like bedtime routines, feeding routines become a critical part of helping your child establish limits and structure.

Family meals should encourage and reinforce the following mealtime parameters:

- Meals have a beginning and an end.
- Eating is social.
- It's okay to be hungry sometimes.
- While we may choose how much we eat, we have to choose from what's available to us.
- Certain behaviors are acceptable and others unacceptable at the table.

Consider these key elements to healthy feeding as babies approach toddlerhood.

SELF-SERVING BABIES | WHEN DOES A BABY BEGIN TO FEED HERSELF?

Most children will begin to show an interest in feeding themselves around nine or ten months of age. You can facilitate this step toward dietary free will by preparing small portions of soft, diced food such as well-cooked vegetables, fruit, or easily crunchable oat ring cereal.

EMPOWERING YOUR BABY WITH STUFF THEY CAN PINCH

Make your pinchable pieces compelling to hungry eyes:

- **Don't put out too much.** Your baby's eyes may be bigger than her esophagus. Limit self-serving to two or three pieces at one time. This will prevent overstuffing and overstimulation.
- **Keep it small.** Pieces should be small enough that a child won't choke on the food if she swallows it whole. Keep food pieces smaller than the width of your pinkie.
- **Offer the spoon-feeding before self-feeding.** Once your

child experiences the novelty of self-feeding, you may find her resistant to the traditional bowl and spoon. If spoon-based foods are on the menu, offer these first and understand that over time the total volume of pureed food will fall off in favor of solids.

SHOULD YOU SEASON YOUR BABY FOOD?

When it comes to adding salt and seasoning to your baby's food, there are a few things to consider.

- **It's not about you.** Parents consistently taste what they give to their babies. I get this. The problem is that there's the urge to salt and season when what we deliver doesn't meet our personal expectations. Don't bring your own perception of how things should taste to your baby's high chair. Babies come into the world quite comfortable with the natural flavors of vegetables until we show them otherwise.
- **Salt should be avoided.** Added salt should have no role in your baby's diet. Your baby needs very little salt, and what she does need will come naturally from her milk and basic foods. As solid foods are advanced, there will be a natural increase in the hidden salt that your baby sees. So no need to add extra.
- **Seasoning is reasonable.** While we have come to expect that baby food is supposed to be bland, the truth is that this isn't the case in many parts of the world, where subtle seasoning in the norm. A pinch of rosemary or a dash of cumin can liven up a boring bowl of squash. However, I would avoid using seasoning to get a child to eat something she might otherwise not be interested in. Instead, I like the idea of seasoning once a child is able to appreciate that this is not the only way a food tastes.

- **Breast-fed babies are tasting from the get go.** Remember that babies on the breast experience a variety of tastes and flavors long before we ever entertain seasoning solids. Breast milk is a natural reflection of what mamma sees in her diet, since many tastes make it through to your milk. The breast-fed baby will grow from her earliest days to expect certain tastes based on a mother's diet.

- **What we deliver will set a precedent for years to come.** Be it the bad habit of supplemental salt or the cultural tradition of spiced apples, what we choose to deliver will set a precedent for years to come. And while cultures vary in their view of spiced foods, the fact is that mashed potatoes are never quite the same once you've had them with a pinch of salt.

SOLIDS AND THE EVOLVING APPEARANCE OF YOUR BABY'S POO

You can't change what you put into your baby without changing what you get out. This is an absolute law of the digestive universe. It's like gravity, but with a unique odor.

Think about it: when you start baby food, you're fueling those hundred trillion inhabitants of your baby's gut lumen with new carbs and substrates. The new sugars and fibers found in her fruits, vegetables, and cereal shift the babybiome. Sure, the key players that make up her microbial footprint (the ones *you* gave her) will still be there. It's just that the supporting cast will change, and as a result you'll notice other changes.

Beyond solids bringing new fuel for bugs, your baby's physiology will also change. For example, the fat composition of a solid diet will change the speed at which things move through the intestine. And beyond the wacky dietary changes your baby undergoes is the fact that her bowel is growing and maturing, as she's no longer in the fourth trimester of gut development.

As one would expect, all these transitions add up to an altogether different number two. While I'd like to tell you not to worry, you will worry when you see how peas and summer squash mash up as a diaper patty.

So, if you dare, look for changes in your baby's diaper.

POO BY NUMBERS

In general, feeding can impact diaper counts in any number of ways. Don't believe anyone who thinks they can tell you how it's gonna go down . . . or come out. Your only saving grace is the reassurance that your baby's stooling pattern may change temporarily while something new is added, but this typically passes within a few days.

ODOR

As a now-almost-seasoned reader of *Looking Out for Number Two*, you know that poo gets its foul odor from the bacteria that live and grow in the colon. As new sugars make their way into the colon and as different types of bacteria grow and prosper, you will notice a significant change in the odor of your babe's poo. This could work for or against you.

COLOR AND THE FRIGHTENING REALITY OF THE UVO

Unless you're picking bananas or looking for shoes to match your bag, color is really just a detail. But understand that your baby's crap can appear in crazy colors depending upon what's eaten, in what combination, and how it's metabolized. We'll go into the deep

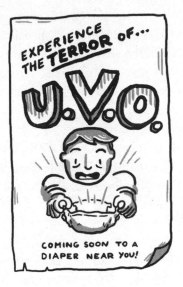

details of poo color in Chapter 7, but sit tight for now knowing that unless it's red, white, or black, the changes you see are of little significance.

And remember that as your baby moves beyond pureed vegetables, it's not uncommon to see UVOs (unidentified vegetable objects) in the diaper.

CONSISTENCY

If your baby's stool consistency doesn't change with solids, I'll refund you the price of this book (be warned that you will have to prove it with a panel of clearly documented before and after diaper shots). This can run the gamut from pellet-like and impossible to pass to loose and slimy.

Of all the changes you'll observe in your baby's diaper, consistency is one that you may need to act on. Loose, runny bowel movements can mean any number of problems. For most babies this means simply that she isn't quite prepared yet to deal with a particular food (simple intolerance). It may indicate an allergic reaction, although in the absence of rash or vomiting, this can be difficult to prove—so be careful about writing off a certain food because of a "reaction" or strange-looking stool. If your child has a runny diaper with bananas, try again in a couple of months when her gut is a little better adjusted.

Hard poos that make your baby strain are common with rice cereal and it may be that you'll need to limit this and other foods that create a problem. Replace cereals with meat to help your child get the iron she needs.

No BOOK ABOUT WHAT COMES OUT OF A BABY IS POSSIBLE WITHOUT SOME discussion of what goes in. Over the past couple of chapters, you've learned a lot about feeding and fueling your baby's growing body and a strong babybiome, and you've seen that food helps fashion the shape, size, and color of your baby's number two.

Speaking of number two, let's get to the meat of the subject with a thorough discussion of what your baby creates in her diaper.

PART II

WHAT COMES OUT

THE ART AND SCIENCE OF
THE BURP

W HAT BETTER WAY TO START A DISCUSSION ABOUT THE STUFF THAT
comes out of babies than with burping? The thing with
burping is that everybody wonders about it but no one talks about
it. Part of this comes from the fact that few of us really understand
it. But when you understand the why and how of this charming
phase of digestion, it begins to make sense and becomes a little
easier to work with.

While we may get into a little navel-gazing here, it's all in the
spirit of knowing a little more about your baby and how her gullet
works. And beyond providing relief and tender loving care to your
precious little bundle of wind, you can use this knowledge to im-
press friends and relatives with your evidence-based understanding of gas.

BURP BASICS

WHY DO BABIES NEED TO BE BURPED?

So here's a core reality of parenting: babies need to be burped. But why? What is it about babies that forces this strange demand to belch? A better question might be: Why do we burp babies but not toddlers? It turns out that when it comes to feeding, babies don't have it all together. This means that the steps that happen to safely get milk from the breast or bottle into the milk hole and down into the stomach aren't all that organized. In fact, you can see it yourself when you watch your baby feed. You'll notice sounds, noises, and a different look coming over them when they swallow.

This comes from a natural degree of discoordination during feeding. As babies protect their windpipe while simultaneously getting milk down the swallowing tube, it isn't a perfect thing. It's almost perfect, but not perfect enough to prevent things from sometimes going off the rails. Feed a baby and you'll see some sputtering and discombobulation every now and then. Listen to a baby feed and you'll hear the sound of gulping as they swallow.

And as they eat they also have to breathe. It's not easy being a baby.

Altogether, the process of suck-swallow-breathe results in air going into the stomach. It's a small amount that goes down with the milk, but over the course of two breasts and twenty minutes, it adds up.

Here's the key point of the chapter: what goes down must come up. And if it doesn't come up, it must go down. This means that the air that goes in needs to come up, or else it will lead to a painfully stretched stomach. What's worse is that if it doesn't come back up, it'll find its way beyond the stomach and into the intestinal track. Then you're in deep doodoo. Or, to be more clear, your baby is in real pain and there won't be much you can do about it. Hence the deep doodoo.

Once milk goes beyond the stomach, the horse is out of the barn.

BURPING AS THE SECRET SAUCE IN FART PREVEN-TION

Having treated millions of babies with excessive gas (okay, thou-sands maybe), I've learned that the majority with painful gas from *below* struggle with gas from *above*. Typically, one of the following is happening: either the baby takes in too much air or there's a failure to free even the small amounts of air that do come in. As I tell our pediatric residents at Texas Children's Hospital: when fix-ing air from below, look from above.

Or in the words of the Urban Dictionary, a burp is a smart fart that took the elevator up.

As a parent you want to work on facilitating smart farts. You can close the book and chew on that for a while . . . or just take my word for it: babies need to be burped.

WHY WE DON'T BURP TODDLERS

A few minutes ago I put forth the deeply philosophical question about why we don't burp toddlers. As you likely know if you've ever been around a toddler, the reality is that they burp themselves. They also take air in when they feed, especially if they're horsing around with their siblings, laughing, making faces, sticking their tongues out, and carrying on at mealtime. They'll swallow air by default. But they learn to push the right buttons to get rid of it. And as you'll learn, they can sometimes push your buttons as a result.

So while we all swallow air, those of us nonbabies have de-veloped the unique ability to facilitate burping. It starts with the sensation of fullness that we associate with air and follows with our intentional ability to use our belly muscles and a little po-sitioning to let it rip. Babies just don't get this yet. They swallow more air than the rest of us, and they need our help to bring it to a happy resolution.

KNOWING EXACTLY WHEN TO BURP YOUR BABY

A baby needs to burp when they've accumulated gas in their stomach. But since you paid fifteen bucks for this book (and I appreciate that!), I'll take things a little further for you.

The problem here is that there's no good way to know when your baby needs to be burped—it's one of parenting's great mysteries. Babies don't come with check engine lights. There is no app (yet) for gaseous distention of the stomach (though I imagine whoever cracks this one will make the short list for the Nobel Prize in Medicine).

But until then, you're on your own. So here are two approaches you might take:

1. LOOK FOR SIGNS

Despite the fact that babies don't appear to communicate in a way that's superobvious, they do a pretty good job of sharing when something's up—and not burping at the right time is usually our failure to hear what they're saying. In this case it will be a matter of you watching and understanding changes in your baby's demeanor and rhythm. You may notice a subtle change in facial expression or head and neck posture, or a slowdown in the pace of feeding.

In these cases, a burping break may be worth a try. You'll know pretty quickly whether your guess was correct, and you'll be able to file these nonverbal cues away in your parental memory.

This idea of understanding your baby's rhythm will recur throughout childhood. So keep your eyes peeled and your mind open, because no one will know your baby like you do. And it's this unique parental insight that serves as the critical first clue in identifying when something's up with a child.

2. BURP BY THE CLOCK

For many parents and caregivers, this ability to read their baby is too much to manage or too unreliable. In those cases you can downshift to a schedule instead. I would suggest breaking halfway through a four-ounce bottle or between the first and second breast. Usually these natural break points serve as a cue for you to give burping a try. For most of us, this is an easier metric to follow.

WHAT HAPPENS WHEN A BABY BURPS | A MATTER OF POSITIONING AND LUCK

Of course, knowing when to burp a baby is one thing, and eliciting that perfect belch is quite another.

Before we dig deeper into how you burp your baby, it may make some sense to talk about what happens when a baby burps. We know that babies like to swallow air and that they're not so good at letting that air out.

When air goes into the stomach, it accumulates into a big bubble. It may start out as tiny bubbles that collect over multiple swallows, but ultimately the air consolidates and floats up while dense fluid and milk follow gravity down.

A MATTER OF POSITIONING . . .

How a baby is positioned determines where that big bubble of air collects.

- If a baby is on her tummy, gas will accumulate at the back of the stomach.
- If a baby is on her back, gas will accumulate near the front of the stomach.
- If a baby is upright, gas will rise up to the dome of the stomach—very close to the valve that lets things in and out.

This issue of where the air collects is key because the only way that air will ever have a fightin' chance to leave the stomach is if it can collect up high near the valve. Part of our job is to help position our baby such that her air accumulates where it can leave.

So positioning is the first step in eliciting a killer burp.

... AND A LITTLE BIT OF LUCK

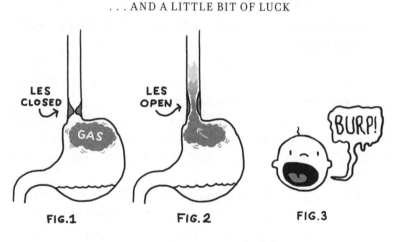

THE ANATOMY OF A BURP

The other key to the killer belch is timing, or luck. Even when a baby is properly positioned, gas can only leave the stomach when the valve—the lower esophageal sphincter (LES)—opens.

As it turns out, the infant stomach is really smart in that it knows that air swallowing is a key issue, and it accounts for that by occasionally opening the valve. In fact, this valve opening happens pretty frequently in babies—on the order of every few minutes. When this quirky little miracle of motility occurs, it's called *transient relaxations of the lower esophageal sphincter (LES)*. I know it's a mouthful and I promise not to say it again. But this is nature's way of facilitating the almighty burp.

Why is this important? We can control a baby's position and where her gas bubble may sit, but *when* the valve relaxes is out of our control. So burping ultimately comes down to luck and a little bit of patience.

A burp, like a really good BM, can take time.

THE ART OF THE KILLER BURP

THE ART OF the killer burp comes down to putting your child in the best position possible, so that when that valve opens, you're ready. So let's talk about positioning your child to burp like a frat boy.

THREE POSITIONS FOR A KILLER BURP

I personally learned how to burp babies from watching the grand masters of burping: the nurses of the newborn nursery. These folks are amazing. They have complete command of the baby—they know when to shift position, how to hold, and how to place that gentle level of agitation that helps gas bubbles get together. The only reason I understand as much as I do about the art of the belch is because I stand on the shoulders of these amazing burp-meisters.

Speaking of shoulders . . . here are the positions that will create the greatest opportunity for your baby to make wind.

OVER THE SHOULDER

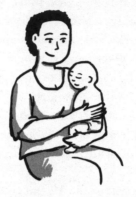

This is the classic burping configuration. Your baby rests against your chest while your forearm serves as a resting place for her bum. Your other hand can rest on the baby's back. Most parents find this appealing because you're chest to chest and your baby's head is nuzzled up close to the side of your neck.

The problem with the over-the-shoulder technique is that when your baby spits up, it runs down your back and all over your ass. Nuzzling is one thing; having a wet, milky ass is quite another.

SITTING FORWARD (SKI JUMPER)

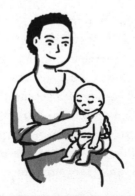

This one is less intuitive for young parents who may not feel at ease putting their child in what may seem to be an unnatural, less-than-nurturing position. What you do here is place your baby on your left knee while supporting her chest with the palm of your left hand. In this position a young baby's head will flop forward. With the thumb and index finger of your supporting hand, hold up your baby's jaw such that her head is tilted up and slightly extended. The forward lurch looks like a ski jumper in flight.

If you've never watched the winter Olympics this may not be the best position for you. Or just consider outfitting your baby with a helmet.

FACEDOWN

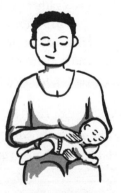

In this configuration you place your baby's chest in the palm of your left hand and hold her facedown. You can rest the lower part of her body over your left knee as you sit. You will need to offer some support to her head with your thumb and index finger like in the sitting forward position. A little subtle bouncing with your hand or knee may help to aggregate gas for that magical moment of valve relaxation.

If you use the facedown position to burp your baby, you'll have to get over the feeling that you're holding your baby like a large piece of produce.

EXPERIMENTATION AND RECOGNITION OF YOUR BABY'S ANATOMY

While I don't want to turn this book into the Kamasutra of burping, you can help your baby belch in a number of creative ways, and it's your job as a parent to find them.

What's key is that all three of these positions put your baby in a different anatomic configuration. The reason this is important is that all babies are made differently, each with slightly different plumbing. So where the gas collects and gathers and the precise angle of the tummy valve varies from baby to baby. You'll find that what works for your sister-in-law's baby may not work for you. Like so much of parenting, you need to experiment and see what's best for your baby.

And when you hit the sweet spot (at the right time), you'll know it. Or, in this case, hear it.

> *A good burp is like porn: you can't really describe it, but you know it when you see it.*

DO BREAST-FED BABIES NEED TO BE BURPED?

If you're like me and you spend your free time reading about intestinal gas, you'll come across the recurring suggestion that breast-fed babies don't need to be burped. I'm not sure where this urban legend got its start, but it simply isn't the case. Breast-fed babies do tend to swallow less air, but they come into the world with the same developmental issues of coordination and control. And while I'm a proponent of breast-feeding, the reality is that babies swallow air at the breast just as they do with the bottle—and therefore they too need help burping that air back up.

WHY DOES TAPPING A BABY'S BACK SEEM TO MAKE A DIFFERENCE?

In my clinic one day, I faced a mother who had just fed her baby and proceeded to rhythmically pat her baby on the back. I innocently asked her why she did that and she sheepishly confessed that she didn't know, but that she had seen it on TV.

Whether we pick up our cues from sitcoms or neighbors, we've all dialed in to the idea that tapping works for burping. And for good reason. Small bubbles of air consolidate to bigger, burpable bubbles with bouncing and tapping.

Rubbing a baby's skin probably has the same effect on burping as standing on one foot or closing one eye. Remember the role luck plays with the relaxation of the LES. If you rub long enough, you just might get lucky.

ERUCTATION (BELCHING) OBSESSION

So what if your baby doesn't burp? This is an important question because some parents are hell-bent on making their baby burp. They believe that the failure to elicit a belch during any given feed will create a nightmare situation, and after all this talk about air beyond the stomach, I get it.

But the reality is that some babies are efficient feeders and don't swallow a lot of air. So their need to eliminate air may be less urgent.

It's also important to keep in mind that some babies are just impossible to burp. Despite your best efforts and ninja capacity for shifting from ski jump to over the shoulder, it just won't happen. Give your baby two to three minutes to burp then change position. If there's nothing there, don't sweat it. Move on to the remainder of the feed or call it a day.

Remember too that if your baby's hungry and screams like a banshee at having the bottle or breast taken away, the amount of air she takes in with all that carrying-on will offset anything you're working to get out. This is a case where knowing and following the rhythm of your baby is a better strategy than anything you'll find in a book like this.

DO ANIMALS BURP THEIR BABIES?

I once sat through a lecture by a pediatrician who suggested that burping was a bad human habit, an urban legend passed through the millennia. His

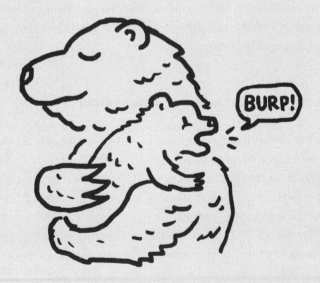

cockamamie theory was supported by one observation: other animals don't burp their young.

While I can't confirm that there *isn't* another
species in the animal kingdom that helps its young
free up swallowed air, it's hardly relevant. Whether
it is or isn't something done by doting mother ba-
boons and bears, human babies like yours swallow
air and need to be burped.

WHEN DO YOU STOP BURPING YOUR BABY? AND OTHER DEEP PARENTAL QUESTIONS

This is one of my favorite questions because if you ask the mothers of, say, a one-year-old when their babies stopped needing to be
burped, almost universally they can't recall. It's something that
typically happens on its own, meaning it isn't something that you
put on your calendar.

One day you'll wake up and you'll realize that you're not burping your baby anymore. More important, you'll realize that she's
no worse for the wear and you'll move on to the next parental preoccupation.

A couple of things will happen in your baby that will make her
independent of your patting and positioning:

- Coordination of sucking and swallowing gradually improves
  to the point where she takes in less air.
- She learns to burp herself.

This will typically happen at some point between six and eight
months of age.

FROM THE MOUTHS OF BABES | SPITS, URPS, AND WET BURPS

I F YOU HAVE A NEW BABY AND YOU'RE NOT FIXATED ON POO, THERE'S A pretty good chance that you're counting how much she spits up. If you're purely a stool gazer, you can skip forward to Chapter 7 where we get down and dirty with number two. Literally.

For now, let's cover the waterfront on what babies come up with.

WHAT IS REFLUX?

ALL BABIES HAVE REFLUX

It happens every day in my practice. A mother shows up with her new baby and asks, "Doctor V, does my baby have reflux?" I always answer without hesitation, "Yes." The reason I can say that with such immediate certainty is that *all babies have reflux*.

That's crazy. How can that be?

Reflux happens when the stuff that's in the stomach comes back up where it doesn't belong. As it turns out, this phenomenon of stuff sneaking up into the swallowing tube happens to everyone throughout the day. It's a common physiologic process. In fact, it's happening to you right now but you probably don't know it.

Reflux shows itself most commonly via spit-up in babies. And when we see normal, physiologic reflux as new parents, we tend to worry about it and wonder what gives.

Since all babies have reflux, the better question might be, "Is my baby sick with reflux or does she have reflux disease?" We'll cover this in just a second.

VOMITING JARGON | LANGUAGE YOU NEED TO KNOW TO TALK WITH YOUR PEDIATRICIAN

There are a thousand words to describe the stuff that comes out of your baby's stomach (and mouth). If you're going to elbow your way into your doctor's office over a pile of dirty burp cloths, you've gotta be able to talk the talk. Here's a primer:

- **Regurgitation.** This word is used to describe the passive flow of tummy stuff up the swallowing tube and out of the mouth. It's usually quiet and stealthy. The typical spitting-up that we see in babies is properly characterized as regurgitation. This is sometimes referred to as spit-up or spits.
- **Urp.** Modern vernacular for regurgitation.
- **Rumination.** This is regurgitation that never makes it out of the mouth. Parents classically "hear something coming up" but never see anything. Rumination can turn into an urp.

- **Reflux.** This is the medical term for regurgitation and some forms of rumination. It's characterized as the presence of tummy contents above the stomach. It's a normal physiologic process that happens in all babies.
- **Reflux disease.** This is when reflux causes a problem like choking, wheezing, screaming, or an inability to feed. It's when the normal, physiologic process of reflux goes off the rails.
- **Vomit.** Vomiting is a coordinated purging of the stomach that involves intense contraction of the stomach, relaxation of the valve at the top of the stomach, opening of the esophagus, and tearing of the eyes. Vomiting is different from regurgitation in that it's an active, reflexive physiologic maneuver to empty the gullet.
- **Projectile vomiting.** Vomiting that's forceful and shoots out of a baby's mouth (often one to two feet) is called projectile vomiting. It's concerning because it can suggest that something's blocked in or just beyond the stomach.

PEAK SPITS | OR AFTER FOUR MONTHS, IT'S ALL DOWNHILL

Baby spits tend to peak around three or four months of age. This may be because a baby's feeding volume picks up ahead of her intestinal motility. The good news is that after this peak at three or four months of age, you're through the worst of it. By a year of age, only approximately 5 percent of babies are still spitting up.

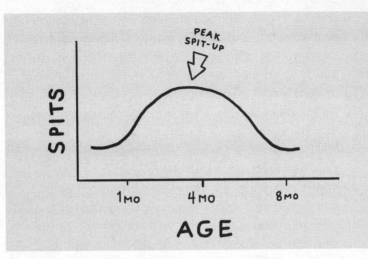

WHAT IS IT ABOUT BABIES THAT MAKES REFLUX MORE OBVIOUS?

You might be saying to yourself, if all of us experience reflux all day long, how come I don't spit up? Or why don't I send my ten-year-old to school with burp cloths?

As it turns out, some things about babies make their reflux more obvious. And the normal, quiet reflux that may only come halfway up *your* swallowing tube may make it all the way up and out of your baby.

Here are a few things about babies that make their reflux more obvious:

- They are on their backs all day long.
- They are on a liquid diet.
- The valve at the top of the stomach likes to open and close.
- Their ability to squeeze and empty their tummy isn't fully developed.

So think about it: when you take someone with underdeveloped tummy squeezing and a loose valve who lies around drinking all day, you've got a setup for the spits. But the good news is that reflux or passive spitting tends to improve partway through the first year. It coincides with the following:

- Development of the ability to sit up
- Advancement onto solid food
- Development of normal tone, or tightness, of the valve at the top of the stomach
- Progression of normal intestinal squeezing (motility) patterns

BABIES ARE NOT LIKE TOILETS

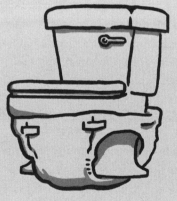

Parents like to talk about the "bad flapper" at the top of the stomach. As it turns out, the valve that separates the swallowing tube from the stomach is a *sphincter,* which is a circular collection of muscles like those around your anus. There is no valve, flap, or flapper. And your baby's anatomy is nothing like your toilet plumbing.

NOT ALL BABIES HAVE REFLUX DISEASE

This is important: although all babies may have reflux, few babies have *reflux disease*. Gastroesophageal reflux disease (or GERD) is when the stuff that normally comes up creates a problem for your baby. This might be choking, wheezing, inability to feed, profound irritability, or weight loss.

For most babies, or even adults, we have ways of protecting ourselves from what comes up into our throat and swallowing tube. Our spit washes it down and neutralizes the acid while our swallowing tube is pretty good at pushing or wringing it back down.

But sometimes our defense mechanisms aren't good enough or the reflux is too severe. In this case, the tummy contents can get into the entrance of the windpipe or even burn the swallowing tube, causing pain and other pesky problems.

IN MY PROFESSIONAL OPINION, YOUR BABY IS A TERD

GER stands for gastroesophageal reflux, or the normal spitting that babies do. We put a "D" for "disease" at the end when that normal reflux creates a problem for a baby. If you dive into the medical journals, you'll find lots of researchers making names for themselves with new acronyms. My favorite is TERD, or tracheoesphophageal reflux disease, which is when reflux gets into the airway.

THE HAPPY SPITTER (OR "I DON'T CARE HOW MUCH YOUR BABY SPITS")

As harsh as it may sound, I don't care how much your baby spits. What I mean by that is that regurgitation alone is not something we worry about or treat. Stuff coming up is less of an issue than stuff coming up and creating problems.

Those babies who spit all day long but who are no worse for the wear are usually referred to in the business as *happy spitters*. The biggest threat presented by the happy spitter is to mom's sanity. The second-biggest threat is to whoever happens to be charged with cleaning the burp cloths.

Don't get me wrong, the happy spitter can generate a frightening amount of recycled milk. But these babies classically show up in the clinic with thunder thighs and more chins than Jabba the Hutt . . . both clear indicators that a baby is getting what she needs.

And nearly every week, almost without fail, I face at least one on-edge mother who points her finger at me and declares, "THIS is not normal." Facing an impending knee to the groin, I typically step back, concede, and agree that spitting up twenty-seven times a day isn't normal. I then qualify, however, that it's *common enough* and *if a baby isn't sick,* we tend not to get excited.

So when do we get excited? Or, more important, when should you consider a decisive knee to the groin if your doctor doesn't seem to be paying attention?

GERBER CLOTH DIAPERS MAKE THE BEST BURP CLOTHS

Take those fancy shmancy embroidered burp cloths from your baby shower and put them away. If you're serious about the spits, you'll use the fluffy, absorbent

Gerber burp cloths from your local baby superstore. They will suck up the spits and protect you from the occasional volcanic eruption that your baby produces.

HOW TO TELL IF YOUR BABY'S REFLUX IS MORE THAN A LAUNDRY PROBLEM

While mild, physiologic reflux is a laundry problem, we can't overlook the symptoms that might indicate reflux *disease* in your baby.

Here are some of the signs that tell us things might be headed in the wrong direction.

CHAOTIC FEEDING

Normally a baby sucks down her bottle or takes to the breast with a peaceful, focused rhythm of suck-suck-swallow-breathe. And as we learned back in Chapter 3, the speed of the feed tells us a lot about how a baby's doing.

As it turns out, when reflux makes a baby's throat and swallowing tube sore and irritated, just having milk go over it can make a baby wince. The way that looks is that your baby will take a few sucks and then arch back and grimace. It's similar to the way you feel when drinking juice with a sore throat.

But as you might notice, the moment your baby pulls off the breast, she remembers that she's still hungry and immediately relatches, only to pull away again. This can change what should be a quiet, enjoyable feeding encounter into a long, drawn-out, forty-five-minute affair.

This chaotic feeding pattern of on and off the breast compounded by the spitting of milk can also lead to poor weight gain. The inability to maintain a normal pattern of weight gain (also known as failure to thrive) tends to get our attention as pediatricians.

UNSTOPPABLE CRYING | "THE BUNDLE OF MISERY"

In addition to poor feeding, stomach contents in the swallowing tube can cause burning and irritation in the chest and throat. Pain such as this can make your baby scream. It can happen anytime, but it is more likely to happen after feeds, when the belly is full and spilling back up into the swallowing tube. Usually, babies with pain from reflux stiffen their bodies and arch with the posture of a world-class diver. There may be head-turning. Picking your baby up to comfort her typically will not make the crying better.

It's a miserable spot to be in for you, and an even worse one for your baby.

DISCOMFORT WHEN LYING ON THE BACK

A baby's pain from reflux may be most noticeable in certain positions. Given the tendency of gravity to pull milk into the swallowing tube when a baby's on her back, a baby with painful reflux may have her greatest pain when she's horizontal or being changed. This positional misery may be better when she's on her belly or upright.

SLEEP DISTURBANCE

Painful irritation when horizontal will create obvious issues when sleeping since babies sleep on their backs. In fact, bedtime may be when they spend the most time in a horizontal position. You may notice what I have come to call "pin-in-the-foot" awakening with reflux. This is the situation where you put your baby down only to have her awaken two hours later with piercing screams representing a painful wave of reflux.

In babies beyond six months of age, this can be mistaken for behavioral awakening (aka, "I don't wanna be alone tonight"), but in those cases babies immediately light up and stop wailing when they see your smiling-but-concerned face.

CHRONIC COUGH, CONGESTION, OR WHEEZING

As reflux makes its way up to where the swallowing tube and airway connect, there can be some spillover into the breathing tube that causes coughing, "choking," and even asthma-like symptoms. Sometimes the generalized irritation of the airway can give a baby noisy, Darth-Vader-like breathing. This kind of breathing is commonly confused with environmental allergies. But if your baby sounds like Darth Vader, it could be reflux. Or she could have gone to the Dark Side.

All casual references to *Star Wars* aside, breathing symptoms can represent one of the most serious signs of reflux disease in babies.

CONSTANT HICCUPS

All babies have hiccups from time to time. Babies with reflux, however, seem to have them all the time. Why babies with reflux are so prone to hiccups is not known.

Having treated thousands of babies with reflux, I've had many mothers tell me that, unlike with their other children, their reflux baby had constant hiccups in utero. This is just an observation, so don't take it to the bank . . . or your doctor's office. But it's an interesting association that comes from being on the front lines of reflux over the past twenty years (it's a dirty job, but someone has to do it).

SPOILER ALERT

It has played out a million times in my clinic. A mother reports screaming irritability when a baby is put down only to be relieved when the baby is held upright. Grandma chimes in with arms folded from the other side of the exam room: "She's spoiled . . . that's what that baby is, (finger jutting) SPOILED."

As it turns out, a twelve-week-old baby lacks the cognitive wherewithal to be "spoiled," and in cases of positional pain such as these, we are sometimes suspicious of reflux. And tough love won't fix reflux.

AND THEN THERE ARE THE GRAY-ZONE BABIES . . .

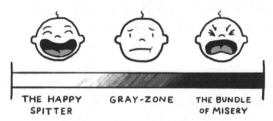

THE HAPPY SPITTER   GRAY-ZONE   THE BUNDLE OF MISERY

As it turns out, spitting may not be all that black and white. It can be gray (or green, as we'll see in a few pages).

Let me explain.

If we took all the babies who live in my community and lined them up in the parking lot of Texas Children's Hospital by severity, there would be a happy spitters on the left and sick kids way over on the right.

In the middle would be our gray-zone babies.

Happy, healthy spitters are easy to identify. Sick, choking babies who can't grow are also easy to pick out. The gray-zone baby in between . . . not so easy.

Gray-zone babies (GZBs) are those babies who have reflux that leads to some of the signs that we listed above, but they still grow well and aren't that sick. They're the screaming bundles of misery who are climbing up the growth curve or the baby who "chokes" constantly but shows crystal-clear lungs in the doctor's office.

These babies have signs that are concerning but they're not quite there yet. They are at some risk since things can turn in the wrong direction while we're not looking. As a pediatrician, the GZBs are the toughest cases since they can slip under the wire and the decisions about treatment can be less than straightforward.

Remember that the GZB can become a sick baby. As parents, we are our baby's only advocate. If there are things that are getting worse and might be overlooked, it's your job to step up and speak out.

> *Reflux, like breast-feeding, is nature's almost-perfect birth control.*

DECODING THE SPITS: WHAT TO EXPECT WHEN THEY'RE SPITTING

Just as there are stool gazers, there are spit gazers. Vomit can create a new obsessive focus that goes beyond poo.

So is there anything we can tell from studying what our babies come up with? Here are a few things to watch out for:

- **Bile.** Bile is a neon-green fluid released by the liver. When we see bile in a baby's throw-up, it can suggest a blockage or partial blockage of the intestine. This exorcist-like output is something that needs immediate attention from your pediatrician or an experienced pediatric ER physician, especially when it's projectile (see below).

- **Clabbered milk.** As it turns out, when the protein found in milk is exposed to acid, it undergoes a change and creates little ball-like pellets called curds. Moms will often call this milk "clabbered." The appearance of this milk is completely normal and is no reason for concern.

- **Blood.** Your instinct is correct, blood in spit-up is never normal. But one of the most common sources of blood in spit-up is swallowed blood from a cracked nipple. The stomach lining in babies can get inflamed, however, and give off a little blood. This needs attention, but a small amount isn't an emergency.

- **"Coffee grounds."** Blood that's been in the stomach a little while can undergo partial digestion and turn brownish like coffee grounds. So this raises the same concern as having blood in the spit-up.

- **Mucus.** Parents often report mucus in their baby's spit-up. The reality is that the stomach creates mucus of its own, so seeing it in vomit is of no particular concern. Swallowed mucus from the sinuses or lungs can also show up in the throw-up.

- **Old food.** Typically, things like milk and baby food should be gone from the stomach within about two hours of eating. This can vary depending upon what your baby eats (fats move out of the stomach slower). Either way, food that's thrown up more than two hours after it's been eaten suggests that there could be a problem with the way the stomach empties or squeezes. Less commonly, it can suggest a blockage, although this kind of vomiting is usually more forceful.

- **Forceful vomiting (aka projectile vomiting).** Vomit that shoots out of the mouth more than six to twelve inches suggests that there's a pretty significant amount of force behind what you're seeing. Typically this suggests a blockage until proven otherwise. Look for immediate attention from your pediatrician or an experienced pediatric emergency physician.

STAND CLEAR: IT'S PYLORIC STENOSIS

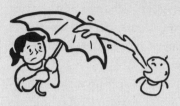

If your baby is around a month of age and has consistent vomiting that shoots out of his mouth almost immediately after eating, your doctor will think about a pyloric stenosis. Pyloric stenosis is a condition where the muscle at the exit of the stomach gets mysteriously thickened such that milk can't pass through into the intestine. Since the exit of the stomach is partially blocked, milk can only go the other way. It's more common in firstborn males and is fixed with a simple operation that opens the thickened muscle.

FIXING REFLUX

NORMALLY, REFLUX IN babies fixes itself. But when it gets in the way of your baby's growth and simple ability to be a baby, there are some things pediatricians recommend.

HACKING YOUR BABY'S REFLUX WITHOUT PILLS AND POTIONS

Sure, there are pills and other concoctions to help control reflux. But what can you do at home to help your baby with reflux? Remember that reflux is an issue of intestinal motility or squeezing. If your baby's prone to it, you won't be able to make it go away, but you can definitely cut into it.

BREAST-FEED

Breast milk is superefficient at emptying from the stomach and represents the best form of nutrition for the refluxing baby. I see this every day when mothers transition from breast milk to formula before going back to work—there's a predictable increase in a baby's spits when the change is made. This effect is not enough to *not* make the transition to formula, but enough to prove the point that breast milk is best for spits, urps, and wet burps.

If you can't breast-feed, keep reading . . .

USE THE RIGHT BOTTLE

This is an issue that's almost never discussed, but it's key. Baby bottle systems allow milk to flow at low rates and high rates. If you're using a bottle system that is on the low flow side and your baby's hungry, she'll suck like crazy and draw in air around the nipple. A rate of flow that's too high will cause your baby to choke, sputter, and (you guessed it) swallow air. All this air will put your baby at risk for reflux. Start with a standard flow nipple and look for a sucking pattern that's quiet, rhythmic, and without dribbling, squeaking, or squawking sounds.

BURP A LOT

While you may only burp your baby once during a feed, another break to curb your baby's air swallowing might help. But also remember that if your baby is a feisty feeder and doesn't appreciate the "break," her screaming may actually worsen the amount of air that she takes in. This is one intervention that you're going to have to figure out based on your baby's temperament.

PUT GRAVITY ON YOUR SIDE

Keep your baby upright for at least thirty minutes after her feed. A chest harness like the Baby Bjorn carrier is a great way to do this while keeping your hands free.

CONSIDER ALLERGY IF YOUR BABY SHOWS THE SIGNS

As we'll learn in Chapter 10, allergy can look just like reflux in a baby. If her spits are connected to constant crying, heavy mucus in the poo, and an eczema-like rash, she may respond to a hypo-allergenic formula (with an extensively hydrolyzed protein). More on this later.

TRY SMALLER, MORE FREQUENT FEEDS

Smaller feeds will definitely make for smaller spits. But remember that you will need to feed more frequently to meet your baby's total daily needs. As we'll discuss next, keeping your baby hungry is not a solid strategy for reflux.

STARVATION IS NOT A STRATEGY | WHY FEEDING LESS WILL NOT FIX YOUR BABY'S REFLUX

As pediatricians, we sometimes blame parents for their baby's problems. And when it comes to spitting-up, it's easy for us to suggest that parents are feeding their babies too much. Blaming reflux on overfeeding takes the doctor off the hook and puts responsibility for the problem squarely on the parent.

But that's not the source of the issue. Remember that reflux is an intestinal squeezing problem, not a feeding problem. Minimizing what a baby eats is never a winning strategy for the spits.

What's more important here is that for a baby with reflux who is consistently spitting up and losing calories, she will likely be hungry and will need to feed more frequently in order to make up for lost energy. I have treated thousands of babies who were restricted in their feeding in order to avoid the inconvenience of dirty burp cloths. Then the parents wondered why their baby was so miserable. Beyond the risk of undernutrition, hunger is a powerful stimulus for crying, air swallowing, and more reflux.

So while smaller feeds are one approach to the spits, you will need to offer those feeds more often so that a baby's daily milk volume is enough to meet their needs for growth and development.

BABIES ARE NOT LIKE KETCHUP BOTTLES | THICKENED FORMULA AND OTHER FOLKSY MANEUVERS

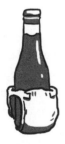

When it comes to managing the spits, I can assure you that you'll be advised by someone to add cereal to your baby's milk to thicken it. If your pediatrician doesn't recommend it, your neighbor will. It's what we've always done because it seems to make sense. It makes sense because if you've ever worked in desperation to get ketchup onto your french fries, you know that thick, high-quality ketchup is hard to get out of the bottle.

So, as the logic goes, thick formula should be hard to get out of a baby.

But while this recommendation would make me look like a

doctor of decisive action, thickening formula doesn't appear to make babies better. A megastudy of studies done by the esteemed Cochrane Group looking at the effects of thickened formula on reflux failed to demonstrate any clear benefit.

And I have to say that in the years that I've been a tummy doctor, I don't believe I've ever had a mother report that her baby was any better with the use of thickened formula. Yet I've never had even one who was unwilling to give it a shot.

I agree that it seems to make sense, but a lot of things that seem to make sense just don't work when it comes to hacking your baby's regurgitation. Maybe because babies aren't little bottles of ketchup.

Still, when you're a parent, sometimes what you believe trumps what's real.

WHAT A TANGLED POO WE WEAVE

The other thing with cereal is that it creates more problems than it's worth. And remember that we're starting with the fact that it's not worth much.

In this scenario, it all starts with the nipple. When you add cereal to a bottle it makes it hard for your baby to get it out of the nipple. So then they suck, pucker, squeak, squawk, and draw in air as they desperately work to get pudding-consistency milk out of a pinhole opening. Then they get pissed off and spit up more because they're hungry and they've got a gullet full of air.

If you make it that far and milk actually reaches your baby's stomach, you'll face the fact that rice cereal potentially creates cementlike stools. So then they grunt, squeeze, and strain desperately to produce a marblelike turd, all the while turning purple, swallowing air, and further increasing their risk for the spits.

And remember that cereal added to formula adds extra calories to what your baby takes in. The reality is that we don't know the long-term effect of supplemental cereal calories in early infancy.

But wait, there's more to this story.

When you drop in to your pediatrician's office with a baby pumping out bricklike turds, he'll give you a medication called lactulose to soften the stools caused by the cereal used to treat your baby (who happens to just be a happy spitter). Lactulose is fairly rich stuff and potentially slows the emptying of the stomach, thereby increasing risk for reflux.

It sounds like I'm making this up, but I see it every day.

So while your mileage may vary, use cereal at your own risk.

TAKE THE CEREAL CHALLENGE

So now that I've made it clear that thickened formula doesn't work and that it instead potentially creates a near catastrophic diaper scenario, let me go ahead and tell you how to go about adding cereal to your baby's formula. This is a little like telling your teenager not to have sex but casually leaving condoms on his dresser.

It's just that if you're gonna do it . . . I want you to do it right (the cereal, not the sex).

Here's my *Number Two* recommendation:

1. **Use oatmeal.** Studies show that oatmeal is less likely to give your baby bricklike turds.
2. **Add one teaspoon of cereal per ounce.** Use the flaked infant cereal that comes in the box.

Go ahead, take the challenge—and as I tell parents in my clinic, I love to be wrong when it works. But if it doesn't work, stop doing it.

I'll add that there are formulas with rice starch built in. The only advantage to these added rice formulas is that the number of calories in every ounce is precisely what a baby needs, which will avoid the risk of overnourishing your baby.

REFLUX AND FORMULA ROULETTE

Since we're on formulas, let's settle a couple of things on milk and spitting.

When we have a screaming, arching, impossible-to-soothe bundle of misery baby, we often demonize the drink. If we just found the right formula, we rationalize, she'd be like the baby on the cover of the magazine.

As it turns out, there are no babies like the ones in the magazines, and, with the exception of the added rice formulas, there are no milks designed to treat reflux. And that makes perfect sense, because as we've learned, reflux is a muscle and nerve issue, not a milk issue.

With that said, there is a big fat hairy exception: the baby with milk allergy, whom we'll talk about in Chapter 10. Milk protein can react with the lining of the intestinal tract and cause all kinds of symptoms like colic, screaming, blood in the poo, eczema, and even spitting. Dig into that chapter for more details, but understand that in those cases a baby must be treated with a hypoallergenic formula.

And to clarify, in those instances we'd be using formula to treat a baby with allergy, not reflux. There are no formulas to fix reflux.

Did I say that already? Some things are worth repeating.

STARTING SOLIDS WILL FIX REFLUX (AND OTHER URBAN LEGENDS)

Parents of babies with reflux often have questions about starting solids. Like cereal (and expensive ketchup), there's the magical belief that heavier stuff will stay put. I tell parents that reflux shouldn't change the way they advance solids in their baby. At the end of the day, some babies will get better on solids, some will get worse, and others will just spit up a Technicolor spectrum of squash and green beans.

REGURGITATION NATION

As you'll read in Chapter 11, when colic was first described in the 1950s it was the hot new thing. And throughout the latter twentieth century whenever a baby cried, she was diagnosed with colic. It was a constellation of symptoms positioned as a diagnosis that had no clear treatment. For better or worse, colic was the label that kept pediatricians free and clear from fixing the problem. There was no fix.

Fast-forward to the early twenty-first century. Reflux is the new colic. Unfortunately, some of my colleagues have fallen into the habit of labeling every inexplicably fussy baby with reflux. What's worse, some act on the impulse and prescribe medications when they're not indicated. Some of this is a function of a new label. Part of this may be a consequence of doctors seeing more and more babies in the same eight-hour clinic day. A label and the promise of a pill have a certain appeal when facing a desperate, tired mom in a six-minute follow-up visit.

So proceed with caution if your doctor hears crying, sees a dirty burp cloth, and immediately wants to start medication. Remember that you are your baby's lead advocate. Take the time to consider all that we've talked about over the past few pages before assuming medication is the only and best solution.

NO. 2 CASE: THE CASE OF THE SLEEPING FEEDER

Austin is a six-month-old with acid reflux that has led to painful, chaotic feeding with pulling from the bottle. Increasingly over the past month, Austin's mother has noticed that he feeds better at night or when he's asleep. While he might normally take forty-five minutes to take four ounces, feeds offered when he is very sleepy go down in ten minutes. In fact, during the day Austin's mother has taken to timing his feeds during his naps.

I like to refer to this as dream feeding, and it's something that I encounter on a regular basis in my pediatric gastroenterology practice. It's a feeding pattern that can develop in babies suffering from gastroesophageal reflux. With ongoing and consistent discomfort with swallowing, babies develop an aversion to feeding. In other words, they associate sucking and swallowing with impending pain. But when they're asleep, they are less aware of what's coming and seem to feed more efficiently. And even after the reflux is gone, the behavioral pattern can persist. This pattern of feeding is concerning and typically requires the care of an experienced gastroenterologist and feeding therapist.

TO MEDICATE OR NOT TO MEDICATE

While some doctors may have abused the reflux diagnosis, the reality is that there are babies who deserve a shot at relief. So who should be treated for reflux? That's easy: babies who are sick. So who's sick? That would be the baby who . . .

- **Can't grow.** The baby who can't drink what she needs or loses more than she takes, resulting in poor growth.
- **Can't breathe.** The baby who has experienced airway problems like wheezing, dangerous choking, or pneumonia.
- **Can't stop.** The baby who is a bundle of misery, as I like to call them. This is subjective because every mama thinks her baby is miserable. Let's just say that babies who are in so much pain from their reflux that it affects their ability to be babies deserve a chance at relief—if the symptoms of reflux fit.

While this may all seem really straightforward, identifying who's sick and who can be watched is the subject of an ongoing debate that I don't intend to settle.

Ultimately treatment comes down to a decision between you and the pediatrician who takes the time to thoroughly assess your baby. This is hopefully a pediatrician who not only recognizes that reflux is a real problem, but is also willing to identify the healthy gray-zone baby who should be left alone.

It's a tough job, this baby business.

MEDICATIONS FOR REFLUX

So how do we treat significant reflux in babies? When it comes to medication, there are two main options.

ACID BLOCKERS

Reflux treatment is centered on acid control, as acid is what creates the irritation and pain. What's important to understand about acid control is that it doesn't stop the reflux, it just helps control the pain that the reflux creates. When babies are truly suffering from acid reflux, these acid blockers are pretty effective at cutting into symptoms.

It's important to note, however, that not all babies spit acid. For years we've assumed that the pain that comes with regurgitation in babies is caused solely by the acid coming from a baby's stomach. But studies have shown that about half of all reflux events in children don't consist of acidic material. As it turns out, other stuff in the intestinal tract can come up too, like digestive enzymes and bile salts from just beyond the stomach. This may explain why some babies with all the classic signs of reflux don't get better when we block their acid.

The challenge is that we can't tell what kind of reflux a baby has just by looking at her, and we don't yet have good interventions for the baby with nonacid reflux.

SQUEEZING MEDICATIONS

If we assume that reflux is a motility, or squeezing, problem in babies, perhaps we can stimulate the stomach and valves to do what they're supposed to do using squeezing (or prokinetic) medications. While this seems to make perfect sense, the medical studies show that their use doesn't impact reflux symptoms significantly.

With that said, I have found there's a group of sick reflux babies who will respond to select medications. So while motility medications are not considered first-line defense and their track record is less than perfect, they shouldn't be totally discounted. We just need to manage our expectations and understand that not all reflux cases can be managed by motility medications.

QUIETING THE BURN WITH A LITTLE MYLANTA
If it looks like your baby's reflux is shaping up to be more than a laundry problem (and you're stuck with an arching, screaming, hiccupping bundle of misery who won't quiet down), a little topical antacid like Mylanta may do the trick to cut the burn. Try one-half teaspoon used a couple of times a day. While it's a temporary solution, it may get you and your baby through the discomfort until you can talk to your pediatrician about other remedies.

TESTS AND STUDIES

Reflux is a diagnosis best made by listening to a baby's story. And while stories are never perfect, they give pediatricians a pretty good sense for what's going on. That being said, when we have a specific reflux question in mind, there are some tests we can do to help answer those questions.

What follows are a few of the available reflux tests, along with some information about when pediatricians tend to use them and other insider knowledge.

UPPER GI SERIES

What is it? In this test a baby swallows liquid that can be seen on an x-ray. The liquid outlines the intestinal tract and allows the doctor to see if there's anything wrong with a baby's anatomy.

When do we use it? When we think there might be a blockage, like with a baby who has forceful vomiting.

What you need to know. It makes zero sense to order this test to look for reflux since all babies have reflux (if you missed this, turn to the beginning of this chapter). This test is often ordered in babies, but it exposes them to unnecessary radiation and is rarely necessary (unless your baby has persistent or forceful vomiting).

PH/IMPEDANCE PROBE

What is it? A test in which we put a tube in a baby's nose to measure acid and nonacid reflux, as well as other things like burping air.

When do we use it? When we want to measure how much reflux there really is or to connect reflux with certain events like coughing or stopping breathing.

What you need to know. This is a great test when you want to connect suspected reflux to some kind of funny behavior. For example, if a baby constantly arches her back and turns her head to one side, the doctors may want to use the impedance probe to connect that funny posturing with reflux instead of, say, seizures. One issue is that it can be hard to keep that tube in a baby's nose.

NO. 2 CASE: THE CASE OF THE OVEREVALUATED HAPPY SPITTER

Savannah is a four-month-old who spits up nearly continuously. The spit-up amounts to frequent "wet burps" of various quantities. During her routine checkup, it's noted that Savannah is a happy, healthy baby who feeds beautifully and is growing nicely at the 90th percentile. Savannah's mother mentions her frustration regarding the spits to her pediatrician, who suggests that they move ahead with an upper GI series and an impedance probe to "see what's going on."

Reflux in babies is a clinical diagnosis. What that means is that we listen to the story and diagnose the problem based on the evident pattern of the baby's symptoms. So happy spitters are quite comfortably diagnosed with a careful history. Remember that all babies can show some reflux, so seeing it on an upper GI series won't help you. And knowing how much is coming up and down from an impedance probe won't make a difference, since this isn't a baby sick enough to treat. This is a situation where understanding and reassurance from your pediatrician will take you, as a parent, a lot further than expensive tests.

ENDOSCOPY

What is it? This is the examination of the lining of the intestinal tract done with a thin, fiber-optic endoscope. Endoscopy allows us to both look with our eyes as well as take small samples to look at under the microscope.

When do we use it? We use it to look for inflammation that may be causing symptoms (allergy, reflux) that are unclear or not responding to treatment.

What you need to know. If your gastroenterologist jumps to this up front, think about getting a second opinion. This normally isn't done unless your baby is very sick or has an unusual story.

It's important to understand that these tests will not fix your baby. When used in just the right way, however, they can help steer a sick baby in the right direction.

THE BOTTOM LINE ON WHAT COMES UP

At the end of the day, remember that all babies have reflux but few are sick with it. And while there may be no magic pill for your spewing volcanic baby, it's likely to be history well before your baby hits her first birthday. Remember as well that between now and then, you can take some simple measures to make it more tolerable for you, your baby, and anyone brave enough to hold her.

In summation:

- Know what's normal and what isn't.
- Use simple measures to control spitting.
- Use medications when reflux makes a baby sick.
- Know it will go away soon enough.

Poo Basics | Understanding Number Two

Diaper backwards spells repaid. Think about it.
—MARSHALL MCLUHAN

WHEN WE'RE WAITING FOR A BABY TO ARRIVE, WE PARENTS ARE made to think about what we're going to put into our babies (breast versus bottle), but no one ever asks us to think about what's going to come out.

Let's take some time to do that now. What is poo and why should we be thinking about it? As we discussed, babies don't appear to do a whole lot. They eat, sleep, and poo. But what they make in that diaper can tell us a lot about their health and well-being.

Here's a brief-but-fascinating dive into what your baby makes and delivers from below.

WHAT IS POO?

First things first. What is this stuff? Well, it's mainly the stuff that can't be used by your baby. What appears in her diaper is

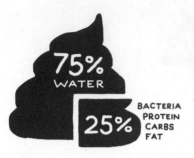

what remains after most of the nutrients, energy, fluid, and vitamins have been removed from her milk. Much of what makes up your baby's poo is water. The rest is a mashup of bacteria, protein, carbohydrates, and fat. Bacteria accounts for over half of the solid part of your baby's poo.

A FEW THINGS TO NOTE ABOUT YOUR BABY'S POO

Here are a few basic poo takeaways:

- **There's lots of water.** This means that as the amount of poo increases, the amount of water your baby loses increases as well.
- **There's lots of bacteria.** The bacteria your baby receives in the early days of her life will shape (quite literally) what she makes.
- **Not everything is used.** Babies naturally fail to absorb some things that they eat. Over time, a baby gets more efficient at removing nutrients from food.
- **Time changes all poo**. As your baby's digestion matures and her diet changes, the makeup, shape, and color of her poo will change and evolve. During the fourth trimester of gut development, the intestinal tract and everything in it grows and changes just like the rest of your baby.

Let's drill down on what your baby's poo will look like during the first couple of weeks of life.

THE EARLY POO TRIFECTA

During the first two weeks of life, a baby will undergo a three-phase shift in elimination, a pattern I like to call the *early poo trifecta*. Or, to borrow from the megaparenting bestseller, this is *what to expect when they're pooping (during the first two weeks of life)*.

1. MECONIUM (YOUR FIRST INITIATION INTO CHILDHOOD)

Meconium is the stuff that comes out of a baby during the first few days of life. It's the leftover gunk from swallowed amniotic fluid and in utero bowel development. You won't miss this because it's greenish black, sticky as hell, and typically requires a jackhammer to get it off your baby's backside. Meconium's single redeeming quality is that it doesn't stink.

2. TRANSITIONAL POO

Meconium disappears after about five days and your baby begins the shift to regular baby poo. But in this in-between stage you have transitional poo—a hybrid of meconium and baby poo. Depending upon the kind of milk you're giving your child, the poo will evolve to look more like that of a formula-fed or breast-fed child (more on what these look like later).

3. BABY POO

At seven to ten days of life, babies will arrive at their baseline baby poo. At this point, your baby has likely settled in with a core population of gut bacteria. This government-issue baby poo is likely what you'll have until you either (1) change milk or (2) introduce solid food. Two things that you will very likely do.

WHEN YOUR BABY HASN'T POOED BY TWENTY-FOUR HOURS OF LIFE

I swore when I wrote this book that I wouldn't fill it with scary crap that puts already nervous mothers further on edge. Unfortunately, raising children comes with some scary crap. Or in this case, a scary lack of crap.

One concern that can arise is when a baby hasn't had a bowel movement during the first day of life. If you haven't yet figured it out, babies are born to make poo. It's what they do best. And when they don't do it, we worry about what could be cookin'.

Failure to pass meconium can be a sign of a problem with the development of the lower colon or a sign of an incomplete opening of the bottom (anus). Conditions like cystic fibrosis are also associated with delayed meconium passage. This is something that your pediatrician or neonatologist will investigate, and usually you can't leave the hospital until it's worked out (literally).

And, for the record, a 2003 study in the *Journal of Perinatology* showed that what you feed your baby (breast milk or formula) appears to have no impact on how soon that first poo appears.

POO AS AN INDEX OF FLUID ADEQUACY

Perhaps the best indicator that a baby is receiving sufficient breast milk is the presence of wet diapers. A breast-fed infant should make six to eight wet diapers in a twenty-four-hour period. Urination tells us that a breast-feeding baby's fluid intake is up to par and that her nutritional intake is most likely adequate. Poo is more variable but can also serve as an indicator of adequate milk. After the first four or five days of life, a breast-fed baby receiving adequate breast milk generates about four stools per day for the first month or so.

POO PATTERNS

EARLY BOWEL PATTERNS | WHAT'S NORMAL

As we learned, the poo patterns of new babies don't settle in until a week or two after birth.

And beyond the evolution of the early poo trifecta, you'll likely find that poo is slow to get going if you are breast-feeding your baby. As you will figure out, your breast milk doesn't just magically appear. It takes a few days for your breasts (and tired brain) to come around to the idea that they need to be making and releasing milk. And during that time period, when production hasn't met demand, things may be slow from down below.

Remember that if there isn't much going in, there won't be much coming out the other end.

THE RULE OF FOURS AND THE FIRST MONTH OR TWO OF LIFE

As a general rule, a breast-feeding baby of a mother making milk will be on the poo bus by around three or four days. If that isn't the case, it may make sense to talk to an expert about what you're producing or how your baby is feeding.

If everything manages to go according to plan from there, your baby will follow the rule of fours. **The rule of fours suggests that after four days of life a baby should have at least four poos a day for the first four weeks.** In fact, I'd expect more like one poo with every feed, but the rule of fours is an easy rule to live by and a great way to help young stool-gazing parents keep track of the absolute minimum. So as we've suggested, things are slow to get moving, but once they do you can expect a lot of dirty diapers.

BOWEL ACTIONS

If you speak with a British accent and do poo re-search, you're likely to refer to taking a dump as a *bowel action*. While I've never fully understood the need for such a formal term, it nonetheless remains de rigueur terminology for those who think about poo and have high-pressure anal sphincters.

WHAT HAPPENS WHEN WE POO? THE BASICS OF THE HUMAN POO PROCESS

To understand the process of how your baby "makes a diaper," it might be helpful to understand what actually happens when we eliminate. While this may seem like TMI, it isn't for a book about all things poo. And this basic understanding of elimination ultimately becomes important for potty training and the speed bumps you might hit later on.

WHAT WE DO WHEN WE POO

Here's how it goes down (or comes out) for the average pooer:

1. **Poo arrives in the rectum.** Through the normal process of intestinal motility or squeezing, fecal matter makes the turn through the sigmoid colon and into the final stretch of the rectum, where it hangs waiting to be expelled.
2. **We sense something's there.** We feel pressure, or fullness, in the rectum and on the pelvic floor.
3. **We hold on until the time is right.** When that fullness sensation goes to our brain, we make the social calculation that the frozen food section where we're standing may not be a good place to do what needs to be done. So we intentionally hold on using our external anal sphincter and some of our pelvic floor muscles to keep things in place.
4. **We sit and let it out.** Actually, it's more involved than that. We sit with our hips flexed. Then we relax our bottom and push with our abdominal muscles to create a little pressure. And there you go.

When all is said and done, we sense that our bottom is empty. We clean up and go on our way. This is the normal, nonbaby cycle of continence and elimination.

HOW YOUR BABY IS DIFFERENT

The poo process for babies is different in a lot of ways. Babies are not cognitively connected to what's going on, or to what's coming out. They can't directly associate rectal fullness with the need to do something else. And despite our upcoming conversation about "potty training" babies, they certainly can't make judgments about when and where to let go.

Babies do learn and understand that the generation of pressure plus the relaxation of the pelvic floor results in a relief of pressure. Beyond this primitive reflexive ability to push, the high amplitude contractions of the colon as well as the gastrocolic reflex (see page 170) play a significant role in moving things along and out.

POSITIONING FOR THE PERFECT POO

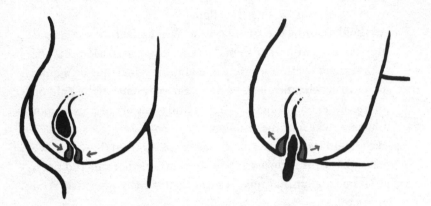

Have you ever tried to poo standing up? Okay, that was a weird question, but it brings up an important point: positioning is important. And as it turns out, for stool to make its final passage into the light of day (or the darkness of a diaper), things have to be aligned just right.

There's a sharp turn between the rectum and anal canal, or the final segment before the anus. When you're out and about, walking and running, this angle plus the job done by the external sphincter muscles helps to keep things in where they belong.

Squatting, flexing the hips (pulling them up), or pulling the legs up straightens out the angle between the rectum and the anal canal, making it easier for the poo to pass. Babies, like dogs, instinctively know this. Or at least they figure it out pretty quickly.

And as you may find out in a couple of years, toddlers who don't want to poop learn that stiffening the legs and arching their bodies and backs is a good way to avoid dealing with number two.

Just remember: **Poo flows best with knees to chest.** And you can't poo standing up.

WHAT IS A CODE BROWN?

If you really want to call yourself a parent, you have to first participate in a code brown. A code brown is a situation where a baby creates a dangerously large mess as the result of a megabowel action. For the purpose of this book, a code brown is typically:

- Initiated by the passage of a large amount of poo.
- Occurs in a situation in which you're unprepared.
- Requires an uncountable number of wipes.
- Involves cursing.

A good example would be a supraphysiologic blowout through the onesie at twenty thousand feet while traveling alone with your baby. Cabin pressure change on the colon can be a bitch.

While understanding the potential for a code brown at any point might be reassuring, keep in mind that it's not a code brown unless you're thoroughly unprepared.

THE BIG SLOWDOWN: BOWEL MOVEMENTS AT ONE TO TWO MONTHS

Your baby will slow down considerably with regard to her elimination between one to two months of age.

Why is this important, you ask?

It's important because if you're keeping track (like a good stool gazer), you may think that something's up. And, in fact, something is up. Your baby's body is changing and her gut is maturing. This is part of the *fourth trimester of gut development* where things are transitioning from life in utero to life in the big bright world.

Why the slowdown? It comes down to the squeezing patterns generated by your baby's enteric brain (those nerves that line the intestinal tract). The rhythmic waves that push intestinal contents on their way move from a chaotic pattern to a slower, more thoughtful pattern. It is quite possible that the evolving maturity of the babybiome is influencing the big slowdown in baby elimination during this period.

Rest assured that this change isn't due to constipation, but rather a normal development of a healthy poo pattern.

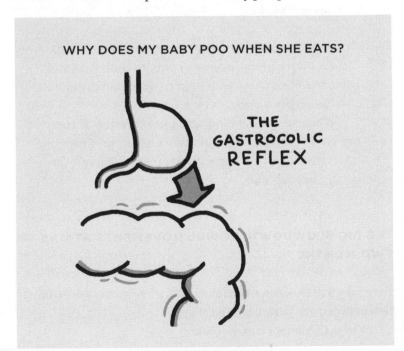

WHY DOES MY BABY POO WHEN SHE EATS?

THE GASTROCOLIC REFLEX

Some things in life are fairly predictable. And one of those things is that after a young baby eats, she'll often poo. Why is this? It's due to a mechanism in the body called the *gastrocolic reflex*. When the stomach stretches with milk, it stimulates the colon to push and squeeze, resulting in (as some of my poo research colleagues like to say) a bowel action.

This effect is more pronounced in some babies than others, and it can even persist into adulthood. This may also explain why Uncle Joe makes a predictable disappearance every year after Thanksgiving dinner.

BREAST OR BOTTLE: WHO POOS MORE?

The gastrocolic reflex explains some of the differences in poo patterns that we see between breast-fed and bottle-fed babies. As it turns out, breast-fed babies poo more frequently than formula-fed babies. In fact, we see about 25 percent fewer bowel movements in breast-fed infants who are supplemented with formula when compared to purely breast-fed babies. Breast-fed babies feed more often, and so the reflexive connection between stomach and colon kicks in more frequently. More feeds means more diapers.

Nutritional factors play a key role as well. Breast milk is rich in nondigested oligosaccharides and protein, which increases the volume, density, and, ultimately, frequency of the poo. On the formula side, the fatty acids and mineral content are higher in formula-fed poo and carbohydrates happen to be lower. These differences can lead to a firmer formula-fed poo and can reduce the frequency of elimination.

As we're seeing, what goes in affects what comes out—which means there's different poo for different milk.

STOOL-GAZING: THE EARLY YEARS

Our fixation on feces has historical precedent. Before medical technology evolved to where it is today, physicians depended on their senses of sight and smell (and even taste in some cases) for diagnosis. Dr. J. Forsyth Meig's 1874 *Practical Treatise on the Diseases of Children* suggested that doctors "ought by all means to inspect personally the appearance of the matters ejected . . . no description of a mother or nurse, however intelligent, can impart to the physician the precise and accurate idea of the state of those discharges which even a very rapid inspection would give him." While I can't imagine examining the stool of every one of my ten thousand patients, Dr. Meig's paternalistic position has given way to a more parent-centered view of baby care. We now trust that parents can make certain judgments on their own.

TMI: REAL ESTATE AND LITTLE ITALIAN POOS

One Italian study demonstrated that poo frequency is inversely related to the number of rooms in a child's house. More rooms, fewer poos. Go figure. It's still unclear whether moving to a larger home treats diarrhea.

FIFTY SHADES OF BROWN | DECODING YOUR BABY'S DIAPER

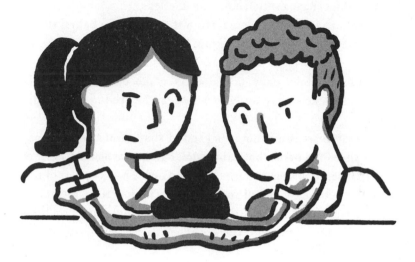

Now that we've covered *how often* a baby eliminates, we'll turn to the next preoccupation of the stool gazer, which is *what poo looks like*.

In some cases, the appearance of a baby's stool can be really important. In other cases, however, stool appearance is just something that fuels parental anxiety and makes them spend money on poo books. So, like many things in parenthood (and pediatrics), the art comes in knowing when to get worked up and when to let things slide. Or plop.

WHY YOUR BABY WON'T CREATE THE PICTURE-PERFECT LOAF

Dr. Mehmet Oz once aired a famous segment where he appeared to divine almost magical health information from poo shape.

From pellets to the textbook S-shaped stool, he had it all sized up. Poo shape is of great concern to stool gazers, and some books on the subject have even become bestsellers.

What can we actually learn from the shape of a baby's stool? I wish there was a simple diagram to connect stool shape with baby bowel health. If there were one, I'd print it right here. But, unfortunately, baby poo doesn't come out in diagnostically predictable shapes and sizes that can be used to predict the future.

One of the reasons that this kind of shape and size prognostication doesn't work is that babies don't make the picture-perfect loafs that we all associate with a trophy turd. The first year of life is a chaotic time for bowel movements. The fourth trimester of bowel development brings all sorts of wild changes in bowel flora and motility patterns, and these changes affect the shape of the outcome as well.

SO WHAT SHAPE SHOULD YOU EXPECT WHEN THEY'RE POOPING?

Your baby is more likely to generate a semisoft mess than anything else. Certainly during the first few months of life, bowel movements are frequent, soft, and relatively small. You're unlikely to see anything resembling a Lincoln log or Baby Ruth bar. There simply isn't enough residual matter in the first months of life to generate the bulk and form necessary for a healthy loaf.

As time marches on, however, what goes in changes, evolves, and ultimately impacts what comes out. Expect more traditional poo to debut sometime during the middle of the first year, in connection with a baby's expanded palate, mature babybiome, and more stable motility pattern.

HOW POO IS LIKE A BANANA, AND OTHER DISTURBING ANALOGIES

When it comes to looking at what comes out of us, hue is important. And knowing how poo gets its wonderful brownish hue helps us understand what's going on when color deviates.

Poo gets its color largely from bile, which plays a critical role in digestion. Bile is made by the liver and then pumped into the gut to help in the digestion and absorption of fats and vitamins.

When bile comes out of the liver, high up in the GI tract and just south of the stomach, it sports a bright, neon-green color. As bile mixes with food and makes its way down the digestive tract, it undergoes a transition in color from green to yellow and, ultimately, to brown, after which it emerges gloriously from the keister. I like to use the analogy of a banana ripening from its inedible green to its almost inedible rotten-brown stage.

Understanding this origin of poo color becomes important when troubleshooting tummy issues in babies. We'll see that when the liver (or the ducts leading out of the liver) doesn't do its job, poo can lose its color. If the intestine is emptying quickly, poo can deviate toward an alarming bright green.

COMMON POO COLORS

Here are some common poo colors:

- **Tan and thick, like hummus.** This is the appearance of formula-fed poo.
- **Dark green.** This can happen with iron supplementation or with hypoallergenic formulas.
- **Seedy yellow.** Breast-fed stools are classically "seedy" yellow . . . like mustard.

WHY ARE BREAST-FED STOOLS SEEDY AND YELLOW?

So we know that breast-fed stools are yellow from bile, but why are they so seedy? Breast milk has a lower protein concentration than formula, which means that it is probably absorbed more completely. This leaves little residue for "stool matrix," or the stuff in poo that glues everything together. As a result, breast-fed stools are more seedy by nature. Breast milk also has a fair bit of lactose, which is slightly malabsorbed. Malabsorbed sugars keep water in the colon making the stools more watery, acidic, and well suited for acid-loving bacteria.

SHOULD GREEN POO SCARE YOU?

Because green poo always alarms the novice stool gazer, it's one of the leading questions parents put to pediatricians. And as I just suggested, it indicates that things might be moving through the digestive tract faster than the bile pigments in the poo can change hue.

In most cases of neon-green poo, we're facing a happy, healthy, bouncing baby. For these babies, their motility (that's the pattern of squeezing) is programmed to move just a little quicker. In other cases, it may represent a gut that's still sorting itself out in the fourth trimester. Think of it as an immature pattern that's maturing into one that's healthy and adapted for the child and adult world. Many of the funny things we see in the first few months of life represent this kind of intestinal sorting.

There's another reason things may move more quickly through a baby's digestive tract. Babies who snack at the breast are more likely to get milk that is predominantly foremilk. That's the thinner, sweeter milk that flows at the beginning of a feed, and it has a tendency to move through the bowel at a brisk clip. The fatty hindmilk slows motility and allows milk to undergo its color maturation as you might expect. While the green poo seen with heavy amounts of foremilk doesn't necessarily mean there's a problem, you can make it go away by allowing your baby to nurse longer on each side to ensure enough hindmilk is consumed.

Often during viral infections such as the dreaded rotavirus, the transit time through the gut can be really fast. So if your baby's electric-green poo comes with a big increase in stool number and a drop in stool consistency, you should be in close contact with your pediatrician. Babies with diarrhea can become sick and dehydrated very quickly.

So when should green poo scare you?

- When there's diarrhea.
- When the amount of poo exceeds what your baby normally makes.

STOOL GAZER ALERT: THREE POO COLORS THAT YOU SHOULD AVOID

You're probably getting the idea that there isn't much to worry about when it comes to poo color. That's the right idea, but there are *some* colors that we like to keep a gazing eye on when they come out of your baby.

In fact, there are three colors that are typically cause for concern: white, red, and black.

Let's unpack these.

WHITE POO

If you've been paying attention up until now, you know that poo gets its traditional color from bile. And when there's no bile, there's no color. Poo professionals and pediatricians call these *acholic stools*. White poo indicates that bile either isn't flowing out of the liver or it isn't being made by the liver. We won't go into the weeds here with liver disease, but understand that white poo in a young baby is something that needs *immediate attention*.

In the interest of full transparency, the white description is a bit of an exaggeration. Poo without bile pigment is actually the color of oatmeal, or really lightly colored scrambled eggs. We don't need to get crazy here with the food analogies, but if there's any question, you should have it checked out by someone who makes a living looking at poo.

RED POO

This one isn't rocket science. As you might have guessed, red poo can indicate blood. Unlike poo that lacks color, blood tends to be universally recognized by those who look after babies and their diapers. The convenient thing about babies is that they don't eat things that are red, so fresh blood is hard to mistake. As you'll learn in a few short months, toddlers like to eat red things. In fact, early in my career Dora the Explorer fruit roll-ups spawned an endless stream of three-year-olds with red poo. But babies don't eat fruit roll-ups, which makes looking at their poo less complicated.

We'll come back to blood in the poo in just a moment.

BLACK POO

So just as bile changes color from green to brown, blood also changes color during its miraculous journey through the gut. Blood that originates way up high in the stomach starts red but undergoes its own digestion and changes to black. Truth be told, the length of the intestines in newborns is short enough and the movement fast enough that even blood from the stomach can make its way through while still red. During its transition, it can sometimes take on a mahogany, bricklike color as well.

And I'll add that before Dora the Explorer fruit roll-ups were wreaking havoc with my mothers, there were those Blues Clues fruit roll-ups which, as you might guess, made poo pretty much black.

NO. 2 CASE: THE CASE OF THE RUSTY DIAPER

Sammi is a nine-month-old girl who has struggled with ear infections. With her most recent infection, Sammi was treated with an antibiotic called cefdinir (Omnicef). Three days into treatment, her mother noticed that Sammi's diaper deposits were a little loose and had a red-maroon color. Concerned that Sammi was bleeding, she took her to the local community emergency room to be evaluated. When the poo was tested, it was found to not contain blood.

As you'll learn when your baby advances on solid food, what you feed your baby can impact how her poo looks. And so it goes for antibiotics and other medications. Cefdinir, the antibiotic used to treat Sammi's ear infection, can generate a scary, red-colored poo. When the antibiotic mixes with the normal iron in a baby's diet, it creates a reddish color that can be mistaken for blood. When the antibiotic is stopped, the color returns to normal.

WHAT TO DO WITH BLOOD IN THE POO?

We sort of glossed right over the idea of blood in the diaper. But the truth is that it's scary as hell for a young mom or dad to find.

It's not supposed to be there, of course, and it always means that something's up.

In the event of blood in the poo, you should consult your pediatrician. The good news is that as scary as it may look, the cause of bleeding isn't serious in most cases. Here are some of the more common sources of blood in the diaper:

SWALLOWED BLOOD

Swallowed blood from delivery or breast-feeding on a cracked nipple can lead to blood in the diaper. Blood swallowed during delivery is typically seen during the first two days of life. Cracked nipples are usually pretty obvious to those who have experienced them. Babies can suck an enormous amount of blood from a sore on her mom's breast. And this blood can be seen in a baby's spit-up in addition to their poo.

Bottom line: Give it time or fix the source of swallowed blood with the help of an experienced lactation consultant. While there are lots of home remedies for cracked nipples, get professional help as this could make or break your ability to breast-feed your baby.

MILK PROTEIN ALLERGY

We'll talk a lot about this in Chapter 10. Until then, know that in about 3 to 5 percent of babies, the protein found in their milk can react with the lining of their intestinal tract and lead to irritation. The blood from allergy typically appears between three and eight weeks of age and is often associated with mucus, colicky behavior, and sometimes a scaly rash.

Bottom line: For breast-feeding moms, eliminate milk protein from your own diet. Bottle-fed babies should be switched to extensively hydrolyzed formulas like Nutramigen, Alimentum, or Extensive HA. Much more on this later.

FISSURE OR CUT

If poo is hard or difficult to pass, it can break the bottom on its way out. While the cut may be tiny, it can lead to a scary amount of blood. Sometimes if you open the baby's cheeks and look right down at their tiny cornhole, you can see a bright red line. But just like cracked, dry fingers in the cold weather, these little cuts can close off, making their identification tricky.

Bottom line: Help your baby soften her poo by giving her two to four ounces of supplemental water or diluted fruit juice. Look out for number two and talk to your doctor if hard stools don't turn soft with the addition of extra fluid.

INFECTION

Just like anyone else, babies can get bacteria in their intestinal tract. While most tummy infections in babies come from people around them, some infections can begin at the time of delivery if the mom happens to be carrying bacteria like salmonella or shigella.

While we don't typically associate viruses with blood in the poo, babies are unique in that they can actually bleed from viruses. Usually the bleeding that we see with both bacterial and viral infections in babies are associated with very noticeable diarrhea.

Bottom line: Infections are often treated with antibiotics, but it depends on the bug and your baby. Since your baby's evaluation will likely involve the collection of a stool culture (a sample to see if bad bacteria will grow), you'll definitely be talking to your pediatrician about this one.

BLOOD VESSEL ABNORMALITY

Babies can be born with little cherry-red blood vessel abnormalities on their skin, which in many cases are more of a cosmetic issue than a threat. But they can also get these small berrylike lumps on their insides. In the gut, where these vascular abnormalities (as they're called) are exposed to acid and digestive enzymes, they can bleed. Usually when babies bleed from this condition there's a lot of blood. These abnormalities are not common and can often be identified because they are associated with corresponding skin lesions. Blood in the poo in any baby with berrylike skin lesions should be taken seriously and checked out by a pediatric tummy doc.

Bottom line: Vascular abnormalities of the bowel are diagnosed by a pediatric gastroenterologist with an endoscope. These may be left alone, treated with endoscopic laser therapy, or sometimes even removed by a pediatric surgeon.

A WORD ABOUT BABIES AND HEMORRHOIDS

After nine months of struggling with hemorrhoids, mothers often rush to judgment and assume that bleeding in their baby could be from hemorrhoids, especially if the baby has a little constipation.

A hemorrhoid is a stretched vein that sticks out from the lining of the intestinal tract or anus. The stretching takes a lot of time to develop and requires pretty serious sustained pressure on the lower intestinal tract. Since babies haven't been around that long, they can't generate the kind of pressure necessary to pop a 'roid. As a result, we simply don't see hemorrhoids in babies.

If you look carefully at your baby's anus, however, you will see little folds of skin that can be prominent. Sometimes babies are born with little "tags" of skin that are mistaken for hemorrhoids. Typically these are very small, they are the color of your baby's skin, and they don't look anything like blood vessels.

Lists of blood sources are nice, but when blood in the poo happens, we have to look at every baby as an individual. We have to think about the bleeding in the context of what else is going on, how the baby looks, how the blood looks, how they're feeding, and how old they are. Blood in the poo is an area where you should get the input of an experienced pediatrician or a pediatric gastroenterologist.

IF YOU DON'T SEE BLOOD, DOES IT MEAN THEY'RE NOT BLEEDING?

This is similar to the old "if a tree falls in the forest does it make a sound" dilemma. The reality is that just because you don't see blood doesn't mean blood isn't there. Blood can be microscopic. In other words, babies can bleed tiny amounts and it may not change the color of the poo. In the trade, we call this *occult bleeding* (and no, it's not associated with witchcraft or wizardry—it just means blood that's not seen by the naked eye). Your doctor might test for occult blood as part of evaluating for allergy, for example.

Occult, or microscopic blood, is discovered using what are called *hemoccult cards*. In this case, poo is smeared on a specially treated card and an agent is applied. If there's blood in the poo, the card turns bright blue.

Nervous moms and dads sometimes read books like *Number Two* and then insist that their baby's poo be tested. Like any test, however, it's important that it be used in a way that's intelligent and useful. As we'll see in Chapter 10, the gut reaction chapter, sometimes we allow a little microscopic bleeding in babies who are otherwise happy and healthy. Again, it's important to understand that what we do with blood in the poo has to be considered in the context of a baby's overall condition.

THERE'S AN APT FOR THAT

Does baby blood look different from mama's blood? To the naked eye, no. Swallowed maternal blood looks just like a baby's blood. But hemoglobin (the molecule in red cells that carries oxygen) is very different between a baby and her mom. Babies have *fetal hemoglobin* and mamas have *adult hemoglobin*. And as it turns out, if you put baby blood and adult blood in separate test tubes and expose them to the chemical sodium hydroxide, the fluid turns a different color. This is called the **Apt Test**, and it's sometimes used to tell a baby's blood from her mother's.

MUCUS, OIL, AND SLIME . . . OH MY

Moving on from blood, another entry in the category of "shit you'll find in your baby's shit" is mucus. Mucus is just what you'd expect—slimy stuff that comes out of your nose or other orifices. A baby's colon makes mucus as a means of greasing the skids for emerging keister cakes. It's supposed to be there, so don't be alarmed. And once your child gets into baby food, her stool can contain derivative products of vegetables and food that can look like mucus (I'm referring again to the UVOs, or unidentified vegetable objects).

But just like your nose makes more mucus when there's a virus making it unhappy, the infant colon can make lots of mucus when it's inflamed. Allergy is the big culprit here. We'll talk about this further in Chapter 10, but usually there are other signs to support allergy. So mucus alone in the face of a happy, bouncing baby shouldn't raise too much concern for you as a stool gazer.

OIL OR GREASE

Oil in your baby's diaper is another story. Often this is really shiny and sits on top of the poo, giving it the unmistakable look of oil. The concern here is that the baby's gut is not doing its part in breaking down and absorbing fat. This can be due to a number of rare conditions, such as cystic fibrosis and diseases of the pancreas, that need thorough attention and evaluation by your pediatrician.

HOW TO GET MECONIUM OFF A BABY'S BEHIND

Meconium is one of the little secrets that comes with spawning another human being. Consider it one of parenthood's foul rites of passage. The big challenge is how to deal with it once your baby passes it. One solution is to prevent its superglue adherence by preventing the sticking to begin with. A small amount of Vaseline, A&D ointment, or olive oil spread thinly around the bottom during diaper changes may make your life easier. After the genie is out of the bottle so to speak, saturated wipes and some old-fashioned maternal (or preferably paternal) elbow grease is your best option.

DIAPERS AND GOING DIAPERLESS

CAN YOU POTTY TRAIN YOUR BABY?

If you spend enough time on the Internet or in certain parenting circles, you're apt to hear about potty training babies.

Let's get something clear. What you will see and read about this trend is not potty training. Potty training requires (1) the capacity to process that there's something in you that needs to come out, and (2) the intention to hold what you've got until you reach a place that's socially acceptable and hygienic to let it out.

Babies lack the capacity to process rectal fullness and, second, lack the neuromuscular wiring to sit and wait for the right time.

Now, with that said, it doesn't mean that when babies need to go they can't do it with the right cue. In other words, if we pay close attention to our babies' patterns of elimination and then use consistent positioning and sound cues at just the right time, our babies can effectively poop on demand.

So to be clear, this isn't potty training or infant potty training, but rather something very different that may or may not be right for you. This has been called *elimination communication*, or EC.

Discerning EC from potty training is important because at some point your child *will* have the capacity to process what's happening down below, and she'll need to connect that feeling with the act of walking to the bathroom, sitting down, relaxing her pelvic floor, and pushing for the end result. This is very different from EC.

ELIMINATION COMMUNICATION ISN'T NEW

Elimination communication isn't a new thing. It's new to some cultures that traditionally have been led to believe that babies can and should only eliminate in a diaper. But during the millennia before disposable diapers, EC was used to minimize the soiling of cloth diapers that invariably fell on the mama's shoulders (or hands) to clean. So I understand the appeal.

Rising concern over the twenty-two billion disposable diapers mounting in landfills has created a new environmentally driven interest in EC. Other parents are driven by the diaper rash that plagues their baby's bottom.

HOW IT WORKS

Although it can be initiated earlier, many parents initiate EC between three and six months of age, and it goes down something like this:

1. **Recognize the pattern.** Elimination communication is just that. It relies on your ability to become superhomed in to when something magical is about to transpire. Facial grimacing, grunting, or straining are common cues for knowing when something's coming. Knowing the pattern of when your baby likes to deliver her keister cakes helps as well.
2. **Provide a receptacle.** Most parents who have successfully adopted EC use one consistent container or pot. With the appropriate cue, hold your baby over the designated container with her hips flexed (remember: poo flows best with knees to chest) and be patient.
3. **Provide consistent cues.** Consistency in cues is key to successful EC. Positioning, holding, and location help. Some parents have made consistent noises that a baby can come to associate with evacuation.

IS EC RIGHT FOR YOU?

Clearly EC isn't something you engage in during a dinner party. Truth be told, it may be hard to entertain at all if you are committed to EC. This can be a messy, difficult process.

Many caregivers keep their children in diapers while learning to connect the dots of elimination behavior and the need to eliminate.

CLOTH VS. DISPOSABLE

Raising babies is full of decisions that make you think. One of those decisions centers around the loin regalia you choose for your baby: Are you cloth or disposable? The argument for disposable diapers is convenience. The argument for cloth is the fact that twenty-two billion disposable diapers pile up in landfills every year.

(Of course, if you use EC with your baby, the point is moot. See above.)

Making this decision can be a lot for new parents worried about when their next four-hour block of sleep might come. Beyond the socioecologic concerns that may come with your decision, there are some other real differences to consider before you go green . . . or plastic.

Cloth diapers are designed for the twenty-first century (sort of). The diaper pins that we see in cartoons have gone the way of the hula hoop. Slightly more chic than the cotton marvels of days gone by, modern cloth diapers are designed to be user-friendly, with Velcro fasteners and crisp snaps made possible through the wonders of plastic.

Cloth: less irritating while at once less absorbent. While the gels and synthetic materials used in disposables may irritate tender young bottoms, cloth diapers are far less absorbent and, consequently, require more frequent changes. Failure to hover means caustic bile acids will have their way with your baby's precious perineum.

Consider the environmental cost of ecologically friendly diapers. While we might feel good about the whole landfill thing, there is the theoretical issue of your cloth diaper's carbon footprint (yes, your diaper has a footprint). Laundering takes water, heat, detergent, and definitely creates waste water.

Diaper service or disposable. It all comes out in the wash. Believe it or not, if you live in the right kind of city you can actually pay someone to clean your baby's diapers. I'm not kidding. Otherwise, you're lookin' at three years of scraping and separate laundering. Disposables will set you back $2,000 to $2,500 a year—about the cost of a diaper service.

There's enough to feel guilty about when it comes to what you do or don't do for your kids. Feeling that you're contributing to the irreversible destruction of the planet doesn't need to be one of them. Do what your bandwidth and conscience allow.

Spoiler alert: I used disposable diapers.

DIAPER STATS

Ninety percent of U.S. parents choose disposable diapers. Their babies burn through an estimated four thousand diapers before they are potty trained.

WIPING YOUR BABY (GIRL)

How you clean your baby is tightly dependent upon their gender. Boys can be wiped any which way. The biggest danger with cleaning a boy lies in the inherent risk of the diaper changer getting a facial shot of fresh, hot urine.

Girls present a more serious scenario, since cleanliness is critical in keeping poo from lingering and getting into the closely approximated urethra, or entrance to the urinary system. The most immediate focus as the parent of a daughter is to see to it that she doesn't sit around in a dirty diaper. Timeliness is key to preventing problems.

When wiping a girl, hold her legs by the ankles and pull them up to expose her bottom. Separate the labia to get into the spaces where rogue bits of stool can sit and linger. Always wipe front to back to ensure that waste is not pulled over the entrance of the urinary tract.

WHAT ARE THOSE CLEAR, GEL-LIKE THINGIES ON MY BABY'S BEHIND?

When you change your baby's diaper you may notice some small, gel-like beads sticking to her bottom. They're alarming because they don't look like something that a human could make. This is just some of the hydrogel that's used in absorbent diapers. These beads pull moisture away from your baby's bottom to prevent diaper rash. The most commonly used hydrogel in disposable diapers is sodium polyacrylate. Sometimes it escapes through the liner surface of the diaper and lands on your baby's skin. It's not absorbed through the skin and doesn't pose any risk to your child.

DEALING WITH YOUR DIAPER

Dealing with what your baby deals out is a major parental preoccupation when you're using disposable diapers. Beyond getting it as far away from you as possible, this is one problem for which there is no solid solution. Assuming that you've dealt with the moral issue of contributing to the global landfill, it really comes down to leaving the diaper in a place that impacts the fewest number of sniffing humans possible.

Foul diapers create an obvious issue for a busy gastroenterology practice like mine. You'd be stunned at the number of folks who pull a dump-and-run maneuver in our clinic rooms. Keep in mind that these diapers represent the worst that babies can deliver—from malabsorption to parasites, dysbiosis to megamethane fermentation. We provide specially designed bags for our parents that, truthfully, don't always do the trick.

The lesson here is that it's impossible to be discreet when you're on someone else's property. Be up front and responsible.

THREE CORE PRINCIPLES OF DIAPER DUMPING

The immediate and timely elimination of your baby's elimination is critical to keeping your nursery from smelling like the ape house at the local zoo.

1. SCRAPE AND FLUSH

The first order of business should be to scrape, dump, and flush diaper cakes in the toilet. While not all parents do this, it's a critical first step in your odor-control strategy. Most harried parents package their baby's stuff into warm, carefully bundled loads of wonder that they dump in the trash can or diaper pail.

2. WRAP AND CONTAIN

Wrap the diaper like a burrito such that the soiled lining is surrounded by the protective outer plastic lining. Use the diaper's tape to create a tightly bundled nugget.

3. DISPOSE AND CONTROL

Dispose of your carefully sealed and contained diaper into a diaper pail. Devices like the Diaper Genie or other equivalent pails allow foul diapers to be hermetically sealed in sausage-like plastic links that can be painlessly dumped on a regular basis. Cost can vary depending upon features and how often your baby fills her diaper. Put a little baking soda in the bottom of the pail and change it whenever you replace your liner.

And one more plug for breast-feeding: breast milk fuels more pleasant-smelling poo. Not a bad bonus.

POO AT THIRTY THOUSAND FEET

If you're stuck beyond the surly bonds of earth, use the air sickness bag found in the back of the seat in front of you. Otherwise, consider traveling with biodegradable dog mess bags that come in a tight little roll. Remember that the FAA does not allow flight service personnel to handle or manipulate your baby's doogie while serving peanuts and club soda.

Your best bet is to discreetly stuff the carefully taped load into your empty Starbucks cup and casually drop it in the bag when the flight service attendant makes her sweep.

WHEN THERE'S NOT ENOUGH POO

Everybody looks at their poop.
—OPRAH WINFREY

F IT'S NOT WHAT BABIES ARE DOING IN THEIR DIAPERS, IT'S WHAT BABIES *aren't* doing that makes us crazy. Straining, pushing, or not making enough poo is a leading preoccupation for the stool gazer.

So how do you separate the grunts from the dangerously concerning elimination problems that keep us up at night? Let's start with the basics of what causes constipation.

CONSTIPATION BASICS

FIRST OF ALL . . . DO WE HAVE A PROBLEM?

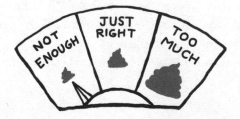

Every day I evaluate babies for different problems. Some of these problems are referred by pediatricians. Others are concerns that parents bring to me on their own. When it comes time to talk about what's going on, the first order of business is to figure out whether something needs to be fixed. If there's no problem, there's nothing I can fix. This is a kind of professional self-preservation.

So job one when it comes to the question of constipation is deciding whether there's something to be concerned about. Because sometimes mothers think that they're facing constipation when nothing is all that wrong. And if we don't have something to fix, we can simply adjust our expectations and go about our business. As we discussed in Chapter 7, a lot of changes happen during the fourth trimester of gut development. If you've got a young baby, you might want to go back there and review what we discussed.

Otherwise, let's talk about the problems that keep your baby from creating the poo that you've always dreamed about.

SO, WHAT IS CONSTIPATION?

Constipation can be defined as a difficulty or inability to pass poo.

But when it comes to what babies make (or don't make), there's a lot of variation. Of course, as we learned in Chapter 7, babies hit a great wall at a month or two of age. For a month they feed and poo. Then BAM . . . we're only makin' one dirty diaper a day.

Even after babies hit their wall, there's a spectrum of individuality in what they produce. Some four-month-old babies poo four times a day, others poo once every four days. And there's the very rare baby who poos every four weeks.

All these examples may be normal. They are reflective of who a baby is and how her motility rolls.

So what do the stats show? This brings us back to the rule of fours. Babies through four weeks should be pooing at least four times a day. After that there's a decline into a pattern that's unique for every baby and her digestive system.

CONSTIPATION IS A PUSHING PROBLEM, NOT A FREQUENCY PROBLEM

What's important to understand is that constipation is a pushing and consistency problem, not a frequency problem. As poo professionals, we get concerned when a baby is simply unable to pass what needs to be passed. And this can happen either when poo is too hard, or when the nerves and muscles can't get it all together . . . or out. In this way, constipation can happen with soft poo, as well.

We'll cover this further in the coming pages. But the main point is that constipation has less to do with calendars or what's normal for your sister-in-law's baby and more to do with what your baby is actually unable to deliver.

THE MARBLE TEST

While constipation is an effort problem, some features of diaper cakes clearly spell trouble and are likely to lead to effort problems. If your baby can pass the **marble test,** she either has a problem or will have one soon.

Criteria for the marble test include turds that:

- Can be picked up and manipulated without getting your hands dirty.

- If not carefully contained, immediately roll out of the diaper, off the changing table, hit the floor, and continue rolling.
- Allow you to reuse diapers repeatedly, as they leave no mark behind.

While poo does not have to be this hard to create a problem, passing the marble test is a sure sign that you need to intervene.

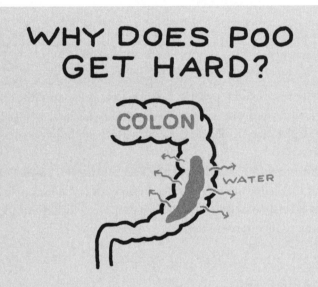

WHY DOES POO GET HARD?

Hard poo is the result of one of two things:

- Too much water removal from the colon (this can happen if poo sits in the colon for too long).
- Nutritional ingredients that set poo up for hardness (soy protein, for example, can make poo hard).

So when we have hard poo, we first think about whether there's not enough water on board, or whether we're fueling the bowel with a food that might make poo concrete-like. More on this later.

BS AND AFTER BS

We can't speak categorically about constipation in babies, since they go through all kinds of different stages of gut maturity and diet in the first year. What's true at one month won't be true at three months and certainly won't apply at seven months.

But one helpful way to think about stool struggles is to look at babies **before BS** and **after BS**. That is, before beginning solids and after beginning solids. When a baby is on breast milk or formula, there are fewer things to think about when it comes to triggers for constipation—and there are fewer creative fixes in our changing table drawer. After BS, there are more places to get into trouble, but more things you can do with a baby's diet.

BEFORE BS: MILK ISSUES

If you chose not to breast-feed or couldn't breast-feed your baby, you may feel bad about the reality that formula-fed babies have a harder time with hard stools. Constipation in breast-fed babies is almost unheard of. In fact, when I evaluate a breast-feeding baby with an elimination problem, I tend to enter the exam room a little bit concerned since the breast-fed baby tends to have a happier lower gut.

THE PROBLEM: SOY FORMULA

In my world, the big bad constipation culprit among formula-fed babies is soy formula, which sets babies up for hard poo. The way that the soy protein intermingles with the fat in formula creates constipation. As you hopefully learned back in the section on what goes into a baby, there's really no reason why any baby needs soy formula.

Consequently, if your baby has a hard time with soy, the first move is to dump it.

USING FORMULA TO FIX CONSTIPATION

Although formulas like soy may set a baby up for hard stools, we don't generally change formulas as first-line treatment for constipation, as there are other things to consider first—such as giving your baby extra water or natural softening agents. But with that said, there *are* formulas that will naturally soften your baby's stool.

Whey hydrolysate. Whey is one of the proteins found in cow's milk. Better known as Gerber Good Start, whey hydrolysate formula makes poos that are soft and easier to pass than standard (casein-based) infant formulas. The broken-down protein leads to a poo with less structure and form. Whey hydrolysate formulas are in the category of standard infant formulas and they taste decent. As suggested, while we don't typically recommend formula changes for constipation, whey hydrolysate formula is a standard infant formula, and a switch to it to potentially make your baby comfortable is not a big deal.

Casein hydrolysate. Casein is the other major protein found in cow's milk. Casein hydrolysate formulas (partially broken down to be less allergenic) are what we call *therapeutic formulas,* and they are used to treat milk protein allergy. Formulas in this category are Nutramigen, Alimentum, and Extensive HA. They smell and they're expensive. Given the expense as well as the fact that we use these formulas specifically for allergy, we don't recommend the use of hydrolysate formulas to treat hard poo.

IRON, INFANT FORMULA, AND THE MYTH OF CONSTIPATION

Any woman who has been anemic during pregnancy has had to live with the constipating consequences of iron supplementation. Iron supplementation can predispose you to painfully hard poo. If you've come off nine months of this, with a raging case of hemorrhoids to boot, you're likely wise to the connection.

This connection has, for years, been carried through to the nursery by mothers who have demanded low-iron formulas, believing that the iron in their baby's formula is a problem. And for years pediatricians promoted the belief that iron in infant formulas could cause hard, painful bowel movements. But this just isn't the case.

Not only does low-iron formula have little impact on bowel movements, it sets babies up for a potentially dangerous iron deficiency that's associated with developmental delay and other issues. Not long ago, after overwhelming evidence failed to show any connection between iron in formula and constipation, the last low-iron formula was removed from the marketplace, never to be heard from again. But I bring this up since it might be something you hear from Grandma.

I've found the best way to explain this to young mothers is that the iron found in infant formula represents the normal dietary iron put there to meet their needs. It doesn't represent "extra" iron.

AFTER BS: FOOD ISSUES

After babies start food, the bowel becomes a totally different world. Bacterial flora change and evolve once they have different kinds of nutrients to munch on. Different nutrients impact motility or squeezing, and the presence or absence of fiber changes everything in the colon.

So while the introduction of foods can set a baby up for hard poo, foods can be used to help turn the whole mess around. It's the blessing and the curse of the after BS baby.

At the end of the day, there's a tight connection between what's in your baby's food and what your baby puts out. Poo in babies is a metaphor for life . . . you get out what you put in.

FOUR TYPES OF FOOD THAT WILL MAKE IT HARD FOR YOUR
BABY TO POO

There are a number of foods that may set your baby up for constipation, but here are a few of my favs:

1. **Rice cereal.** This might be a before BS issue since a lot of parents add cereal to bottles to combat the spits. As we learned, this comes with a price. If it doesn't help your baby's spits, you should stop it. If you feel compelled to add something, consider a switch to oatmeal, which has been proven to improve cereal constipation.
2. **Bananas.** Usually babies will get this through baby food, although quartered banana slices make really nice finger foods to pluck off the high chair table. It's likely the pectin and starch (especially in the less ripened bananas) that can create problems with constipation.
3. **Milk and Cheese.** While milk and cheese may not play heavily during the early months of feeding, you're likely to venture

into this territory after about eight months of age, when your baby starts to experiment more widely. For babies under a year, cheese and yogurt can set them up for constipation. And when your baby transitions over to cow's milk at a year, the risk of constipation rises considerably. Milk protein and calcium come together in the most unique way to create pellet-like or Georgia-clay-like poo (for Yankee readers, this means superdense and almost sticky).

4. **Carbohydrates.** As a general rule, crackers and crunchy snacks can bind up the after BS baby. We've all fallen into the trap of allowing our kids to graze on savory crackers that do a remarkable job of keeping them quiet. But these snacks also tend to quiet the ability of the colon to do what it needs to do. Limit the carbs and crunchies to keep the colon from getting glommed up.

WHEN IT COMES TO CONSTIPATING FOOD, YOUR BABY'S MILEAGE MAY VARY

The problem with baby books is that we like to put little people into tidy boxes with regard to what they'll do, how they'll eat, how they'll poo, and just about everything else. The reality is that what your baby does may be very different. So much of parenting is a string of individual, personally executed experiments where we learn what does and doesn't work for our kids as individuals. Such is the case with baby-binding foods. Your mileage will definitely vary.

NO. 2 CASE: BELIEVE IT OR NOT . . . TWO DIRTY DIAPERS A MONTH

Brittany is a three-month-old breast-fed baby who only poos twice a month. Despite dirty diapers that seem to coincide with the cycles of the moon, she's as happy as a clam. Poos are soft and effortless. Her worried mother took Brittany in to her pediatrician who was equally concerned. He sent Brittany along to a pediatric gastroenterologist, who found nothing at all wrong with her.

This may seem like a crazy example, but it happens more than you'd think. Some babies have a pattern of elimination where they dirty a diaper once or twice a month. These are typically breast-fed babies and the only people who seem to have a problem with this pattern are the mothers and sometimes the pediatricians. Admittedly, the story is unusual, but it represents the variation in the way babies process breast milk. The most important thing is that we have a happy baby with soft, effortless poo. As we like to say . . . this is a baby who hasn't read the textbook.

GRUNTING BABY SYNDROME (GBS)

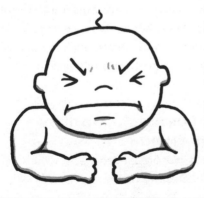

Effort and straining doesn't always represent a problem for babies.

Sometimes issues with passing poo can come down to simple coordination. And if you've ever watched a baby, you know this is something babies don't always have a lot of.

Allow me to introduce you to **grunting baby syndrome**

(GBS). It may be the bane of my professional existence, but it isn't found in the major pediatric textbooks. It's the source of stress and confusion for so many young parents, and too often it's misunderstood if not mismanaged. This is also referred to as **infant dyschezia** by number two professionals.

The baby with GBS will push, squeeze, grunt, turn three shades of red, and carry on—only to produce a soft bowel movement. Parents will then report that their baby is constipated and seek help. Despite the fact that the poo isn't hard, babies often end up on stool softeners, which can make them more uncomfortable. Then we're led down the primrose path searching for a solution.

But in these scenarios, there is no problem.

The grunting baby's problem is one of primitive incoordination. While we all take for granted our understanding of the need for simultaneous relaxation of the pelvic floor and abdominal pressure to poop, not all babies have this figured out. And it's this lack of coordination that makes us believe that our babies are in trouble, when in fact they simply have GBS.

SENSITIVE LITTLE SOULS WITH SENSITIVE LITTLE HOLES

It's important to know that everyone grunts when they poo. When you've got a bunch of waste that needs to come through a small hole, you've got to generate a certain amount of force to make the passage. It's just the way it is. But some parents have a hard time watching their child have a normal bowel movement. In fact, we're witnessing a generation of young parents with no tolerance for any level of discomfort, strain, or conflict in their children.

While no one likes to see anyone suffer, it's

important to understand the difference between straining to poo and the inability to poo. Straining can be a normal, physiologic process that results in a dirty diaper. The inability to make a diaper is just that. Know the difference and don't be a weenie.

STIMULATION ADDICTION AND OTHER DANGEROUS POO GAMES

A common trap for parents and even pediatricians is to stimulate the GBS baby with a thermometer or a cotton swab. When the anus is stimulated, babies exhibit what's referred to as an "anal wink." When this happens, the bottom relaxes ever so briefly, but it's just enough to allow rectal contents to be eliminated.

The reason this is a trap is that it actually works. And because it works so well, young parents will do it again and again. But as the baby becomes accustomed to pooping with stimulation, it comes to be that the baby can only poop when stimulated (thus the trap).

The baby with GBS is best left to work out her issues on her own. The simple timing of elimination is something that we all sort out early on, and we should do our best not to interfere. As difficult as it may be to watch, the short-term relief with rectal stimulation is never a good long-term solution. In my experience, this habit often starts with the recommendation of a well-intentioned pediatric phone nurse who never intended for a parent to do it every day.

SUPPOSITORIES AND STICKS AS SURROGATE STIMULANTS

Beyond the thermometer, there are other things that tweak and tickle the bottom that can get you into trouble over time. Suppositories—little slippery things that go in a baby's bum and stimulate the rectum to squeeze—are a big culprit (see the sidebar). While they can get you out of a bind when your baby's bound, they can be habit forming. They're fine and safe in isolated circumstances, but they should only be used occasionally. Beyond stimulation addiction, glycerin can be irritating to the baby's anus over the long run.

You may catch wind of sticks and wands and other newfangled solutions that help your baby pass gas. It's the same principle of inducing musculature relaxation: okay here and there, but not a good long-term play.

DOSING GLYCERIN SUPPOSITORIES (IF YOU MUST)

While I'm not crazy about suppositories, they play a role. And it makes sense to help you do it right rather than shut them down altogether. It's similar to the issue of teens and contraception—we can't stick our heads in the sand.

For the *occasional* use of treating hard, impacted stools, glycerin suppositories do a great job. Use a standard over-the-counter pharmacy issue adult suppository and cut it in half with a knife. Hold it in your fingers for several seconds to allow it to melt just a little bit. Then pass it into the bottom with your thumb.

In addition to the tickling of the anus, the lubrication and stimulation of the glycerin will often get you—and your baby—out of a bind.

STIMULATION DETOX

Parents of babies with GBS who have fallen into the trap of continuous bottom tweaking leading to the failure of a baby to poop on her own often show up on my doorstep for help. For the GBS baby who can't poop alone, I usually recommend the following.

MAKE SURE THAT THERE'S NOTHING ANATOMICALLY WRONG

This usually involves a teeny-tiny rectal exam to make sure the opening is okay. Your pediatrician or poo expert should be able to take a history and examine your baby to establish that there are no nerve or muscle problems in play.

REMOVE STOOL SOFTENERS, FIBER, AND OTHER "AIDS"

Usually softeners are blindly started without any consideration of what's happening with a baby. And usually these things will make the GBS baby feel worse. Remember that GBS is not the result of poo that's too hard.

TAPER THE STIMULATION

In my clinic I will put these babies on a progressive program where stimulation is withdrawn. So if a mother is stimulating with a thermometer and lubricant every day, I will have them decrease to every other day for two weeks. This allows the baby to decompress and the mother to adjust. After two weeks, I instruct the family to cut the stimulation to every three days. Usually by the time we stretch the stimulation out three days and longer, the baby sorts the issue out and falls into a happy, healthy rhythm of bowel actions.

LET THE BABY PUSH

The tough part for young parents is watching the baby do the hard work of working all their poo out during the days with no stimulation. But this is how the baby learns to relax and push at the same time. There's nothing you can do for your baby except to give her the opportunity to get it done. Despite the temptation to move in and help, this is one thing that your baby will have to figure out on her own.

Spoiler alert: this theme of letting kids work things out on their own will play itself out over and over during the course of the childhood and teen years.

WHY DOES SHE POO WHEN I WIPE? (AND OTHER STRANGE PARENTAL TRICKS)

Here's a variation on the theme of stimulating the bottom in order to get a poo.

Parents learn pretty quickly that the anal wink can be used to their advantage with the grunting baby. On the changing table, they find that firm, aggressive pressure on the anus with a wipe produces a poo. The stimulation of the anus elicits a reflexive relaxation of the external sphincter and facilitates poo passage. But parents will often deny that they're stimulating, since they don't realize what they're doing. Don't fall into this trap.

NO. 2 CASE: THE MYSTERY OF THE BATHTUB POOPER

Ethan is a ten-month-old who has struggled recently with hard poo. The transition from his early-stage baby foods to simple table food has proven too much for him. A penchant for crackers and yogurt has only made matters worse. Poos have been met with crying, straining, and even occasionally blood when the turds get big. Ethan's mother has noticed recently that during his evening bath he will poo in the water.

Older babies, especially toddlers, who have had some experience with painful elimination will learn to hold back when it comes to letting go. Like the little babies who we "potty trained" back in the last chapter, some will begin to learn to associate poo with impending pain. For these babies, the warm retreat of a soapy bath will often allow them to let their guard down and passively relax their bottom muscles. A stealth turd can pop out, creating a water-based code brown. While we should see this as a good thing (getting it out), it often represents a baby who needs a little help.

BATTLING BABY CONSTIPATION

SUPER SIMPLE SOLUTIONS FOR SOLID POO: FIBER, FLUID, AND FRUIT

Here are a few simple things you can try to help facilitate soft poo in your baby.

FIBER

Fiber for constipation. It's the mantra we hear in parenting magazines and pediatrician offices. And for good reason. Fiber stimulates bowel squeezing and offers turds seriously healthy form. But the reality is that fiber can be a huge challenge during infancy. It may be difficult to get substantial amounts of fiber into your baby through her first foods early on. Once you're on to more advanced solids, you may be limited by what your baby is willing to accept. In other words, she may thumb her nose at your bran nuggets. Fiber in toddlers is an even tougher proposition, given their propensity for brazen nose-thumbing and obsessive fixation with a limited number of foods (which are invariably constipating).

If you live with an open-minded, adventurous older baby, the best fibrous foods for fixing firm feces (say that five times fast!) are the following:

Pears   *Prunes*   *Peaches*   *Plums*

Remember, though: fiber without fluid makes cement. And while fiber is important, fluid will get you further.

FLUID BEFORE FORMULA

In the before BS baby, my go-to solution for hard turds is fluid. For the average eight-week-old baby drinking, say, twenty-two ounces of standard infant formula, I recommend supplementing with three to four ounces of water per day as a supplemental bottle. This is usually just enough liquid for the colon to create the mushy consistency that allows things to pass.

The only concern with supplemental fluids is if your baby is having a hard time gaining weight. In this case, putting zero-calorie water in the gullet will take up space that could be used for calorie-rich milk. If your baby's struggling to gain weight, you should probably have a conversation with your pediatrician, as it may make more sense to use a stool softener that takes up less gut real estate.

DO BABIES NEED EXTRA WATER?

You're likely to hear that babies get everything they need from breast milk or formula. But I suspect that the people doing this training have never raised a baby in a tropical environment. In my clinic in The Woodlands, Texas, the temperatures can get crazy high. And when out and about with a baby, the expiratory loss (from heat and sweat) just going from a grocery store into a car can be significant.

Feel free to exercise your parental privilege by offering a supplemental bottle of water in those circumstances when it's really hot or dry. Keep in mind that water in the stomach takes up space that would normally be occupied by milk, so only offer it under really warm circumstances.

When babies lose fluid through their skin, they'll work harder to make up that fluid from places like the colon. Remember that the colon's job is to capture and collect the extra fluid in the intestinal tract before it reaches the butt hole. And so a dry, thirsty body makes for a dry colon—and one prone for pellet-turds.

FRUIT JUICES

Fruit juice represents a more exotic, less-than-healthy way to deliver fluid. Prune juice, for example, contains sorbitol, which has a supersoftening effect. Be warned that babies can become accustomed to the taste of what they get. Fruit juice may contain vitamins, but extra vitamins likely won't do your baby much good as what she really needs is to get her nutrition from breast milk or formula. While prune juice carries a stellar reputation for relieving firmish movements, it's likely that any juice will do the trick. Don't obsess about this. Some juices will also contain fiber, but again, it's likely the hydrating effect of the drink that will bring the turd home.

Like water, the problem with juice therapy for constipation is that there's only so much room in the tummy. And a belly full of juice is less likely to have room for nourishing breast milk or formula. At the end of the day (literally), it comes down to how much milk or formula your baby has consumed. Or, more important, has she grown on a normal curve.

BE CAREFUL WITH NONTRADITIONAL SOLUTIONS

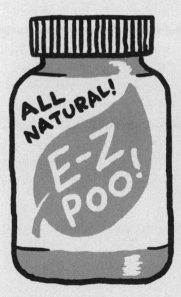

"Natural cures" for constipation aren't hard to find. Just as there are crazy herbs, teas, and drops that you pour into your own colon, you'll find that similar remedies are available for your little bound-up bundle of joy. As a general rule, I would strongly recommend avoiding these quick fixes. Just because it's labeled "natural" doesn't mean that it's something you should give to your baby.

SHOULD YOU CHANGE FORMULA TO TREAT CONSTI-PATION?

While pellet-like turds don't meet the strict criteria for formula change, I certainly won't judge you for doing it. The most constipating formula is soy. Keeping in mind that there really is no clear reason to use soy formula to begin with, switching back to a standard formula would represent the first move.

Otherwise, whey hydrolysate formulas (Gerber Good Start) have been shown to deliver softer, easier-to-pass stools. Hypoallergenic formulas like Nutramigen, Alimentum, and Extensive HA will also give your child softer stools, but other, more conservative measures would be recommended before making the investment in high-dollar hypoallergenic milks like this.

Some formulas containing **prebiotics** have been shown to produce soft turds. Prebiotics are nonabsorbed substances that help promote good bacteria (think fertilizer for good bacteria). Breast milk comes with its own built-in prebiotics—namely fructo-oligosaccharide (FOS), which may contribute to the unique consistency of the breast-fed baby's stool. One formula (Enfamil Reguline) is produced with galacto-oligosaccharide (GOS) and polydextrose, two prebiotics shown to soften stools. And as previously mentioned, the human milk oligosaccharide 2'FL was recently added to several Similac formulas.

Beyond soft, supple poo, babies fed milk with GOS have been found to enjoy levels of the almighty bifido bacteria that match the levels found in breast-fed babies. Wow.

BABIES SOMETIMES NEED HELP BEYOND FIBER, FLUID, AND FRUIT

Here's a reality: some babies need help with number two. It's just the way it is. But that isn't necessarily cause for concern. If your baby suffers chronically with hard poo, it's important to understand that very few dangerous medical conditions predispose a baby to hard, difficult-to-pass poo. Ultimately, it comes down to too much water absorption from the colon or constipating stuff in the diet. Or maybe a little bit of both. And in some cases you simply can't get things in check with extra fluid or changes in the diet. That's okay, and as you'll see next, you can try some other options instead.

DECODING LAXATIVES AND STOOL SOFTENERS

We throw words like *stool softener* and *laxative* around like it's nobody's business. Even as doctors, we say one thing and mean the other. So let's clear the air. When it comes to poo and things we give our babies to help it move along, it comes down to a limited number of things.

STOOL SOFTENERS

Examples of stool softeners commonly used in babies and children include Miralax and lactulose. These hold water in the poo and make it easier to pass. Miralax should only be used on a physician's recommendation and lactulose requires a prescription.

BULKING AGENTS

Bulking agents are essentially a fiber such as psyllium. These add bulk, which can naturally stimulate motility, or squeezing of the colon. Typically, though, our approach to treating constipation in babies is to soften the stool with the products listed above. Fiber doesn't tend to play a big role in treating baby constipation.

STIMULANT LAXATIVES

Laxatives stimulate the squeezing or pushing of the intestinal tract to force the issue of elimination. The bottom line is that you should shy away from using stimulant laxatives in babies unless dispensed by a number two professional. They're usually not necessary, and (as we learned previously) the problem with things that stimulate the bowel is that babies can become used to having that intestinal stimulation. This makes it hard to stop it.

"THIS IS NOT NORMAL"

I've had many mothers look me straight in the eye (and maybe point a finger) and tell me, "This is not normal. A baby should not need to take stuff in order to have a bowel movement." This is a common response when I recommend that we help a baby with a stool softener.

And they're right, it's not "normal." But it's really, really common.

What's important to understand is that constipation is not forever. While babies may go through a period where they need help, it's typically not something that will follow them into childhood. Changes in diet, intestinal bacteria, and motility align to bring babies back to a natural norm. So the things we use to bridge them to that natural state are just temporary measures to get them through. In the meantime, don't sweat the small stuff.

A FEW NON-MEDICAL WAYS TO STIMULATE YOUR BABY

Beyond diet and stool softeners, there are a few other things you can try to help ease a baby's constipation:

- **General movement and play.** Any kind of movement or activity will leverage gravity and potentially create tummy pressure, which helps bowel activity.
- **Hip flexion and bicycle legs.** Put your baby on her back, hold the lower legs, and simulate bicycle pedaling movement. Remember that beyond the stimulating effect of movement, hip flexion creates that perfect angle for poo passage.
- **Tummy massage.** A gentle massage of the left side of the abdomen may stimulate the colon just enough to initiate some squeezing. Starting with some gentle pressure on the upper left side of the tummy, gently massage downward toward the legs.
- **Warm bath.** A warm bath will relax the bottom and pelvic floor muscles such that things may come out more easily.

A FEW THINGS TO AVOID IN YOUR CONSTIPATED BABY

- **Stimulant laxatives.** Medications like Ex-Lax help the bowel push. We generally don't give babies medicines that make the bowel push, as the bowel can get used to them.

- **Enemas.** Even enemas for kids can be too much for a baby's bottom. While we use them in some circumstances, seek professional counsel on this one.
- **Too much poking and prodding.** Along the line of enemas, even suppositories beyond the occasional tweak can spell trouble. If you need to stimulate your baby to poo, you need a different solution.
- **Excessive fruit juice.** It doesn't take too much juice to make things soft. And a baby can have too much of a good thing. Especially when that good thing can cut into what a baby takes from the bottle or breast, and when it creates big gas and, potentially, diarrhea.
- **Mineral oil.** This old-timey stool softener works like a charm, but with babies who spit the risk is too high, as mineral oil in the windpipe can create a dangerous form of pneumonia.

THINGS THAT BABIES ARE BORN WITH THAT CREATE POO PROBLEMS

Babies are supposed to be happy, healthy, and normal. But, unfortunately, babies can be born with things that can keep them from doing what needs to be done. I don't want to make every parent who reads this crazy with fear, but it's important to realize that there are serious things to look for and think about when it comes to babies and their poo.

ANAL STENOSIS

What is it? Basically, the anus is just too narrow.

How is it diagnosed? By rectal exam. If your doctor can't get her pinky into your baby's bottom, that may be a clue.

What do babies look like? Typically babies with anal stenosis push and push and push only to create an explosive, sometimes small, liquidy poo. Sometimes the poo can be pencil-like. This problem can look a lot like grunting baby syndrome (GBS).

How is it treated? Usually with little plastic dilators that you push in to stretch the opening of the anus. In more advanced cases, an operation is needed.

ANTERIORLY PLACED ANUS

What is it? This is when babies are born with their anus too far forward. This makes it very difficult for poo to pass during the final stretch of the colon.

How is it diagnosed? It's diagnosed by looking at the location and proportions of everything under the hood. If your pediatrician produces a tape measure to measure the distance between your daughter's anus and vajayjay, don't be alarmed.

What do babies look like? They typically have difficult-to-manage constipation.

How is it treated? It is usually treated with stool softeners unless it's severe, in which case it may necessitate an operation where the anus is moved toward the back.

HIRSCHSPRUNG'S DISEASE

What is it? This is a condition in which the nerves that help the bowel push never fully migrate all the way to the bottom. This lack of wiring creates a segment of bowel with no movement, so everything backs up.

How is it diagnosed? This can be diagnosed with a biopsy of the bottom that looks for nerves, or a special enema x-ray where a particular pattern is seen in the colon.

What do babies look like? Often babies with Hirschsprung's don't pass their first bowel movement in the first twenty-four hours of life. Otherwise, babies have severe constipation and sometimes poor growth.

How is it treated? The piece of bowel with no nerves is removed by a pediatric surgeon and connected with the bottom. Most babies do just fine afterward. It has no impact on ability to potty train or poo later in life.

HYPOTHYROIDISM

What is it? Hypothyroidism happens when the thyroid (for a variety of reasons) doesn't create enough thyroid hormone. Thyroid hormone happens to be important for bowel motility, so a lack thereof can lead to constipation.

How is it diagnosed? With a blood test. There would also be findings on a baby's physical exam to support hypothyroidism.

What do babies look like? Thyroid disease can affect all organs of the body. Babies may not grow, and sometimes they'll have coarse hair.

How is it treated? Treatment is with thyroid hormone supplementation.

CYSTIC FIBROSIS

What is it? A disease where the glands in different parts of the body fail to secrete fluids and electrolytes in just the right way.

How is it diagnosed? Genetic screening or a "sweat test." During a sweat test, little electric wires are placed on your baby's skin and sweat is electrically stimulated and tested for salt concentration.

What do babies look like? From the gut perspective, they may not poo on the first day of life; otherwise they may struggle with constipation or repeated lung and sinus infections.

How is it treated? It depends upon the type of mutation causing the CF (there are many mutations causing different forms). Usually supportive care of the bowel, supplementation with pancreas enzymes, and special nutritional attention helps babies grow and achieve their normal potential.

SOME SHAPES WORTH PONDERING . . .

If you weren't obsessed with what your baby's poo looks like, odds are you wouldn't have bought this book. And I really want you to think that you got your money's worth, so allow me to feed your obsession. Let's talk a little bit about what poo looks like in babies facing constipation, and what it may mean.

POO IN BALLS

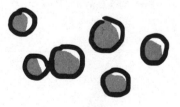

To start, please reference the marble test on page 195. But if your baby's poo appears in little balls, this usually means she needs extra fluid. Two to four ounces of water or diluted juice may do the trick. While often the most painful type of poo, this is typically the easiest to fix.

MONSTER POO OF DESTRUCTION

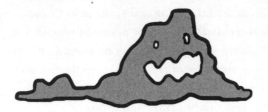

A big poo means that poo is being stored for too long. Your baby can only make so much poo, so when it's big, it typically means that the big poo is actually representing two or three regular poos stored up for a monster delivery. We typically don't recommend that babies deliver three poos at once. Months of constipation in an older baby can lead to a dilated colon that stores poo and facilitates this kind of frightening experience.

The good news is that when big poos come out, we can comfortably rule out a lot of the anatomic problems that lead to constipation, like anal narrowing.

SUPERNARROW PENCIL POO

I never like to see this because it often points to a bottom with a narrowing issue. When the hole is small, all you can make is supernarrow poo. Talk to your doctor or a pediatric surgeon.

SMEARS, SMUDGES, SQUIRTS, AND LEAKS

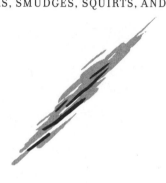

Especially in older babies and toddlers, smears, smudges, and leaks can support the idea that there's a massive backup of poo. In this situation, stool may "leak" around the blockage and ooze out into the diaper, creating the appearance of continuous poo or diarrhea.

DESPITE DOING EVERYTHING RIGHT, SOME BABIES ARE PRONE TO PUSH

Some babies are just prone to hard poo. This may be the result of a colon that's superefficient at sucking out water. It may represent an inherent motility pattern that's a little slower than the average bear. Having treated thousands of bound-up babies, the reality is that at the end of the day, some babies just struggle with poo. And it's these babies who may need support beyond the basics of extra fluid and diet.

When There's Too Much Poo

Changing a diaper is a lot like getting a present from your grandmother—you're not sure what you've got, but you're pretty sure you're not going to like it.

—JEFF FOXWORTHY

DIARRHEA BASICS

DIARRHEA AND OTHER PROBLEMS OF POO VOLUME CONTROL

Diapers with solid poo that can be contained in a tight little taped-up disposable nugget are enough for most parents to deal with. But when something like diarrhea helps stool exceed the boundary of the diapers we've provided for our kids, it can make everyone miserable.

And when mama's not happy, nobody's happy.

Beyond the selfish perspective of cleanup is the reality that something could be wrong. Diarrhea is not normal, and it's one of those clues that something is cooking in the gut. Remember: babies don't appear to do much, so we have to look at what little they actually do in order to see if something could be up.

So we need to take diarrhea seriously. But here's the problem: we don't know what diarrhea is. Let me explain . . .

DIARRHEA—IT'S IN THE EYE OF THE BEHOLDER, OR HOLDER

One of medicine's dirty little secrets is that we have a hard time deciding what diarrhea really is. If you go through the medical literature, you'll find that nobody can exactly agree on how to define it. In fact, if you review studies over the past twenty years, you'll find several different definitions for diarrhea.

And if the diarrhea experts can't get it together, it's unlikely that we will here. But let's not get into the weeds on this one. Let's call diarrhea a pattern of elimination where poo is *increased in volume* and *decreased in consistency*. In other words, when there's more of it and it loses its firmed-up consistency, let's just agree that's diarrhea.

HOW MUCH POO IS TOO MUCH POO?

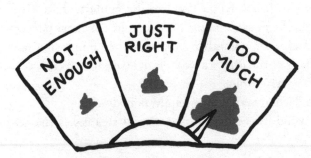

So how much poo is too much poo? Great question because when we look at newborn, breast-fed babies, they poo a fair amount. In fact, they tend to decompress at every feed. If I weren't someone who spends a lot of time thinking about poo, I might think, *Wow, that's a lotta poo!* But when we understand that this is what we expect during the first few weeks of life, it becomes the norm.

Understanding your baby's norm, or her patterns, is key. And it's the recognition of when things change that's going to help you understand when things have gone off the rails. Beyond the absolute definition of what diarrhea is at one point in time, the most important thing to recognize is the change in your baby's poo pattern with regard to amount and consistency.

I've had mothers of breast-fed babies approach me with their healthy, mustardlike diapers and ask me if their baby has diarrhea. This seedy, almost-runny appearance is normal. So in this case, I just say, "That's totally normal," and they go on their way with a new set point of what's normal. Admittedly, stool-gazing's hard sometimes, and you've got to depend on your personal network of other breast-feeding moms or your trusted provider to get that set point.

LOTS OF POO FROM LITTLE BABIES—WHY IS THIS A PROBLEM?

Knowing when things are changing in the diaper is key for the stool gazer because poo patterns are often the first thing to change when a baby is facing a threat from the inside. And when poo volume picks up, fluid loss picks up as well, and a baby can be at risk for getting dehydrated.

The truth is that a three-month-old baby who begins with

liquidy poo due to, say, a viral infection can get dangerously dry within a few hours. So seeing the pattern is key to intercepting a dangerously sick baby. This can happen quickly, so it's important that you keep your eye on the ball . . . or the poo.

WHY BABIES GET DIARRHEA

When we think about diarrhea, we focus on whether it's acute or chronic diarrhea. Acute diarrhea is diarrhea that is relatively new. Chronic has been going on for over three to four weeks. While *Looking Out for Number Two* doesn't intend to prepare you for certification by the American Board of Pediatrics, it's important to have some feeling of whether your baby's poo problem is an everyday thing or whether it's something bigger.

INFECTION

When we think about *acute* diarrhea, the big kahuna is *infection*. In fact, very little else will take your four-month-old baby with daily semifirm, yellow-brown bowel movements and turn her into a ten-stool-a-day, neon-green pooper. There just isn't much beyond infection that will create this kind of mess and threat. Speaking of neon-green poo, when you see that plus watery/runny poo, think infection.

When we talk about infections in babies and children, we're almost always talking about *viral infections*. Bacterial infections can account for the acute onset of runny poo, but it's far less common. Babies tend to be sicker than just diarrhea when they have bacterial infections as well.

If your baby has this kind of acute change in poo pattern, she should be evaluated by your pediatrician or an ER provider comfortable with really small people (see my advice on poo experts at the end of this section).

ANTIBIOTICS

Say your baby needs to be on antibiotics. Depending on the particular antibiotic she happens to need, it can have all kinds of crazy effects on her gut. Some (like erythromycin) will stimulate squeezing of the intestines that will likely make your baby cramp. Others can irritate the lining of the stomach and create painful gastritis.

But the big impact that you're likely to see with an antibiotic is *dysbiosis*. That's a big word for the disruption of the babybiome. Remember that your baby has set populations of different bacteria that live in happy, healthy harmony in her gut. When you knock off a few of the good guys, it creates a critical vacancy that other, less-friendly bugs can populate. In this way, antibiotics create a microbial power shift of sorts. And when bad bacteria have their way in your baby's bowel, they wreak havoc by creating toxins and other by-products that cause inflammation and fluid leakage into the gut.

We call this antibiotic-associated diarrhea, and while antibiotics typically cause acute diarrhea, the changes in the babybiome can alter the bowel pattern for weeks. It's best avoided rather than treated, so don't use antibiotics unless you really need them. Turn to Chapter 12 for more on what you can do specifically in the event that your baby needs to take an antibiotic.

PROTEIN REACTION

We'll dig deep into allergy in Chapter 10, but just remember for now that diarrhea due to allergy tends to be the creeping, chronic kind. You're more apt to see a slow increase in poo frequency and decrease in consistency over a matter of several days. In fact, if you expose your baby to a new protein (the stuff that creates allergic reactions), the kind of reaction that we see in the gut can take a few days to kick in. Usually we also see other signs of allergy like irritability, blood in the poo, and sometimes an eczema-like rash.

TOO MUCH CARBOHYDRATE

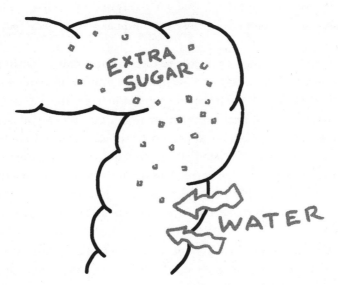

The carb term gets thrown around often in adult exercise and nutrition circles, so when I mention it to parents about their baby they get confused. But your baby actually consumes carbohydrates. In fact, there are carbs in her breast milk and formula.

These carbs tend to exist in certain forms and amounts that are digested and absorbed without a hitch. The problem comes when a baby intakes more carbs than her body can handle. Sugar and carbohydrate absorption happens as milk, fluid, and food slosh down over the lining of the small bowel, and enzymes digest and absorb those sugars. But as it turns out, our body has the capacity to process only a certain amount of these sugars. When we exceed what the baby bowel can absorb, the rest goes downstream and lands in the colon. While some of these calories can be used for energy in a really cool, baby-specific digestive mechanism called *colonic salvage,* extra carbs in the colon can otherwise create the runs.

Carbohydrates can cause acute diarrhea in two ways:

1. **Carbs feed the bugs.** As we learned in Chapter 2, the colon harbors some one hundred trillion bacteria. When carbohydrates are not absorbed up in the small intestine, they make their way down into the colon and those hungry bugs have a party. They create gas, acids, and other stuff that causes diarrhea.
2. **Carbs hold the fluid in the colon.** Sugars that head downstream increase the concentration, or richness, of what's in the intestinal tube. This density, or *osmolarity,* tends to hold more water in the colon and make poo runny. In fact, we leverage this fact in babies who have constipation due to pellet poo. When we add the medication Miralax, for example, we are adding stuff to the intestine that can't be absorbed. So water comes to meet it and the resulting poos are soft, smooshy, and pleasing to pass.

Too much carbohydrate in the intestinal tract can come from juices late in the first year. A little diluted juice on the order of two to four ounces a day shouldn't create problems for most babies, but be careful beyond that.

If you are using powdered formula and you are not mixing it according to the directions, the concentration can give your baby the runs. So avoid juices (if you must, no more than two ounces per day) and make sure that you are prepping your powdered formula in just the right way.

NUMBER TWO PROFESSIONALS

When it comes to poo issues in need of a doctor's attention, you should seek out a trained poo professional, someone who makes a living understanding the comings and goings of the baby gut. Here are the players you should trust with your baby:

Pediatrician. Your pediatrician should be your first stop for poo issues. Pediatricians are trained to deal with the common core issues of what goes in and what comes out of a baby.

Pediatric gastroenterologist. Pediatric gastroenterologists are pediatricians who deal with issues related to the gut. They train for three years just like general pediatricians but go on for another three years to learn specifically about the gut, liver, and nutrition. Your pediatrician will usually refer you to a gastroenterologist when there are tummy or poo issues that go beyond the basics. Pedi GIs, as they're called, are the idiot savants of poo and elimination. It's what they think about in the shower (I know, because I'm a pediatric gastroenterologist).

Pediatric surgeon. Pediatric surgeons work closely with pediatricians and pediatric gastroenterologists to handle things that need an operation. From appendicitis to blockages, the pediatric surgeon knows baby plumbing better than anyone.

- **Pediatric radiologist.** Pediatric radiologists specialize in the imaging of babies and children. From x-rays to ultrasounds, MRIs, and CAT scans, they know how things are supposed to look. Pediatricians, gastroenterologists, and surgeons depend on radiologists to apply the latest and greatest imaging modalities to look at what we don't know and can't see.

What's important to note here is that among the number two specialists, there are no doctors who treat adults. Trust your baby's intestine and elimination issues to a board-certified pediatrician or pediatric specialist. Make no exceptions.

WHAT TO DO WHEN YOUR BABY HAS DIARRHEA

WHEN YOUR BABY HAS BAD DIARRHEA

Let's talk about how to handle acute diarrhea. That's diarrhea that wasn't there yesterday and is definitely there today. It's big volume with loose consistency, and usually there's a virus behind it. Here are a few things to keep in mind:

Get professional input. When it comes to babies and diarrhea, you shouldn't fool around. Or, as they say on TV, don't try this at home. The first order of business is to get the input from a trained baby professional. Losses from a sick intestinal tract can add up quickly and exceed what a baby takes in. **Pack the power of Pedialyte.** One way to keep your baby hydrated is with the use of an oral rehydration solution (ORS).

Pedialyte is one of the most commonly available solutions for keeping babies hydrated when they're sick. Pedialyte may save your baby from an IV and a hospital crib.

What's so special about Pedialyte and other rehydration solutions? Won't diluted juice do the trick? As it turns out, electrolytes like sodium and potassium are pretty important in helping fluids move from the gut into the body. There are special molecular pumps that bring in fluid when these electrolytes are absorbed. Pedialyte is specially balanced to deliver just the right amount of electrolytes to help fluid absorption. And it also includes a little sugar to provide some energy for stressed intestinal cells.

In developing countries, rehydration solutions are a baby lifesaver since access to IV fluids can be limited. **IV fluids and bowel rest may be necessary.** When losses exceed input, sometimes we put the bowel to rest so it isn't stimulated or fueled with more liquid-pulling carbohydrates. Sometimes we will give a baby nothing to eat and support them with just an IV until the diarrhea subsides. Otherwise, we can do this by diluting a baby's formula in half with water to make it easier on the gut. Typically, this is something that's necessary only for a couple of days, until the gut can hold its fluid—but the other reason we limit this to a couple of days is because it cuts into a baby's intake of protein, fat, and calories.

At the end of the day, your most critical role as a parent is to recognize when things are headed south, and then seek the number two professional who is going to get your baby back on track.

HOW TO TELL IF YOUR BABY IS DEHYDRATED

Babies are tricky when it comes down to the physical signs of getting dry. They don't do things like big people, so it's important to know *where* and *what* to look for. And while trained poo professionals should have their eyes on a baby with diarrhea, there are things that you can look for on your own as well.

Fewer wet diapers. Babies who are getting dehydrated pee less, and that will mean fewer wet diapers. Unless you're counting diapers, this one may catch you by surprise. Just like poo, this comes down to knowing your baby's normal routine and how it's changing.

Won't blow bubbles. While babies can't really blow bubbles very well, one sign of hydration is wet lips that, with a little wind behind them, can create itty-bitty bubbles. When a baby is dry, this won't happen. In fact, the lips and tongue will look tacky and dry.

No tears when crying. Just like the inability to blow raspberries, the failure to mount a proper crocodile tear can be a solid sign of dehydration in babies. But remember that while babies are born with the apparatus to pump out tears, don't count on them until one to three months of age (in other words, don't count on a lack of tears as a sign of dehydration during the first few months of life).

Sunken soft spot. You've likely run your hand over your baby's soft spot while shampooing her hair. Or maybe you haven't; a lot of parents feel that the soft spot shouldn't be touched, or they freak out at the idea of running their hands over it. You need to get over this and get to know your baby's soft spot (or anterior fontanelle, as we say in the business).

Normally, this squarish region near the front of the top of the head is pretty flat and in line with the bones around it. But the soft spot will sink or become depressed when babies are dry. This is something to look out for in babies under nineteen months of age; around or after that time, the soft spot closes.

Irritability. Babies don't have a lot of ways to tell us when something's up, but irritability is one of them. Irritability is that crazy, inconsolable state beyond fussiness. And in the context of some of the stuff listed above, it can mean your baby is getting behind the eight ball with respect to fluid. On the flip side, though, dehydrated babies may also be sleepy or lethargic. Look for either of these states in conjunction with some of the warning signs above.

ADDING INSULT TO INJURY TO KEEP BABIES HYDRATED

One of the traps that parents fall into comes from the fear of dehydration. When we see diarrhea, we "push fluids." And when we push fluids, we tend to push sugary fluids. But what we feed a baby often exceeds her gut's capacity to absorb it. So our efforts to hydrate can sometimes fuel diarrhea long after the gut has begun to heal itself. I have treated babies and toddlers two weeks out from an acute viral infection only to find that the cause of the diarrhea is diluted apple juice taken in volumes. As it turns out, we can create diarrhea to prevent the danger of diarrhea. Go figure.

POOS THAT EXPLODE (AND OTHER THINGS THAT GO BUMP IN THE NIGHT)

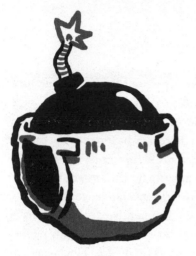

Poos that explode sometimes need a thorough medical evaluation. Usually parents are clued in to the occurrence of high-velocity, exploding stools based on the sound coming from inside the diaper. And if your timing is bad and you catch the bowel action during a diaper change, it can create a critical code brown situation involving your arms and the nursery wall.

Whether you see it or hear it, this sonic boom poo can resemble the action of a sawed-off shotgun: loud, powerful, and with wide-range damage. And as dramatic as that may sound, it's not necessarily all bad.

There are a couple of things to think about with a baby who has explosive poo.

GAS

For the majority of babies, a case of power-loaded poo is the result of gas. Swallowed air or air produced by rogue bacteria build up at the tail end of the colon. When the force of baby's abdominal pressure exceeds that of the internal and external anal sphincters, a bolus of stool followed by a powerful head of steam/air emanate from the anal canal, creating a high-velocity stool.

While sometimes cute but often annoying, baby gas and the ensuing shotgun poo is typically fixable. More on this in

Chapter 11, but as a spoiler alert: swallowed air can come from excessive crying, a poor latch on the breast, or disorganized feeding from something like reflux.

BLOCKAGE

More concerning than the gas-pressure-stool trifecta is the idea that something more sinister could be in play. Whenever a baby consistently experiences this kind of explosive, liquidy poo, we have to consider the possibility that there may be too much pressure for that baby to overcome. In other words, there may be a critical narrowing at the anus that sets the baby up for the situation.

More than a gas problem, the baby with a blockage is typically more miserable and their pattern is consistently explosive. This is something that is first identified with a rectal exam by your pediatrician or other neighborhood poo professional. Most blockages can be fixed by slowly stretching the bottom using little bottom dilators.

NO. 2 CASE: BOTTOMLESS DIARRHEA

Jacob is a seven-month-old who picked up a nasty case of rotavirus diarrhea. After three to four days of really bad diarrhea that required bowel rest and fluid support with Pedialyte, he was advanced back to his regular baby food diet. Though the horribly watery diarrhea disappeared, Jabob's poo continued to be loose and more frequent than normal for him two and a half weeks later. After three visits to the pediatrician for "ongoing diarrhea," Jacob's parents are ready to move on and find a pediatrician who will fix their baby's problem and get rid of his virus.

As it turns out, rotavirus is a particularly bad vi-

rus. It can cause a lot of bowel irritation and injury that can make babies supersick. The fact that Jacob was cared for without ever needing to see the inside of a hospital is a testimony to his parents' care in keeping him hydrated and his pediatrician's good judgment. What's important to understand with viral illnesses is that the tender tummies of a growing baby are particularly sensitive to the insult that comes from big bad viruses like rota. In fact, at this point three weeks after the onset of his illness, his virus has long been eliminated.

What Jacob is dealing with is the residual irritation and altered motility pattern that comes with this kind of infection. This hangover effect can cause poo to remain loose, frequent, and not quite back to normal for up to three or four weeks after an infection like this. Assuming that the diagnosis is correct (and the poo test for rotavirus is good), it's unlikely that another pediatrician is going to endow Jacob with his healthy baseline diaper droppings. If, however, his pediatrician is unable to or unwilling to take the time to explain this prolonged recovery process, that alone may be a reason for his parents to go elsewhere for Jacob's care. As I've learned from twenty years of clinical gastroenterology, it's more about connection and communication from a doctor than it is supersmarts.

Beyond avoiding excessive sugar, there's not much in this baby's diet that will have a big impact on poo consistency and number. As we'll see in Chapter 12 when we discuss probiotics, Jacob might enjoy some benefit (shortened duration of diarrhea) from a probiotic such as *Lactobacillus GG* or *Lactobacillus reuteri.*

DIAPER RASH | MORE A POO PROBLEM THAN SKIN PROBLEM

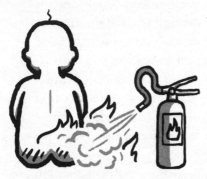

We can't have a conversation about poo without talking about diaper rash. The two go together like peas and carrots (and speaking of peas and carrots, the foods we serve may do their part in bottom breakout). When we think diaper rash, most parents think skin, when in fact they should be thinking poo. If your baby poos, you're likely to encounter diaper rash. If she poos a lot, you'll encounter a lot of diaper rash.

Here's the skinny on diaper rash.

WHAT'S BEHIND THE GARDEN-VARIETY DIAPER RASH?

Irritation. This is reason number one for diaper rash. Both stool and urine contain stuff that irritates and burns the bottom. Burning bile salts that come from the liver are terribly irritating. Bile composition can vary from baby to baby, and this may explain why some babies have burnlike rashes despite the most careful bottom care.

Contact reaction. This is different from the chemical irritation of bile salts and urine. This is an actual contact reaction. Wipes, detergents used for cloth diapers, onesies, or even disposable diapers have to be considered as potential causes of the irritation.

Friction. Diapers that are too tight or too tight at the wrong spot may create just enough chafing to cause diaper rash. When in doubt (and while unfashionable), err on the side of blousy diapers or shop for brands that better suit your baby's unique bottom anatomy.

Yeastie-beasties. Diaper rash that just won't go away should raise a red flag for yeast infection. Often yeast likes to take up shop in the chubby groin folds. It usually looks like red raised pimply spots in the creases, and the spots (or satellite lesions) spread away from the folds. Oral antibiotics can promote the growth of yeast.

New foods. Remember that the introduction of foods puts new things into the gut. These new things find their way out and onto the skin, where they can create a source of irritation. New foods also change the bacterial composition of the colon, which can be another reason for rash.

TREATMENT AND PREVENTION

Keep them dry. Frequent changes represent the best front-line defense to diaper rash. During an active flare of diaper rash, a hair dryer on a warm setting may do the trick to help keep things dry. You can also use small amounts of cornstarch to deal with residual moisture. Apply a small amount to the skin before rediapering.

Pat, don't rub. Friction only adds insult to injury. Pat your baby's bum dry after a thorough cleaning.

Avoid wipes that have alcohol or perfumes. If you're in the throws of a full-blown breakout, wash your baby's bottom after diaper changes and consider pat drying with cotton balls. If you're using cloth diapers, double rinse them to eliminate contact with chemicals and detergents. I would recommend unscented, non-alcohol-containing wipes in this situation.

Go free range. Goin' commando may represent your baby's best chance of maintaining a dry bottom. A bare bottom is a breathing bottom. My grandmother told me that the sun gets rid of everything. While we don't need sun necessarily, you get the picture.

Watch the sequence of food initiation. You'll be able to see the connection between the initiation of a baby food and a new rash, since things move through babies pretty quickly.

Avoid excessive carbohydrates. Remember that supplemental juices, even when diluted, deliver sugar to the colon, which can compound diarrhea and serve as a primary food source for hungry bacteria.

Gut reactions | Allergy, Intolerance, and Things That Go Bump Inside Your Baby

Trust yourself. You know more than you think you do.
—BENJAMIN SPOCK

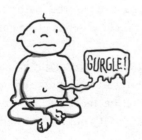

L ET'S TALK ABOUT THE PROBLEMS THAT can happen with the stuff your baby eats and drinks—specifically, the reactions that occur where milk meets the stomach. Parents often fixate on the idea that their baby is reacting to what they're eating, so let's try to separate hype from reality.

As we've learned so far, a lot is happening inside of a baby's tummy. With every new bite of food, babies gain immune "experience" about their environment and different foods. But being presented with all these new foods can actually cause problems. Although babies can react in many ways to these problems, most gut reactions show themselves as allergy, intolerance, gas, or changes in poo—so let's start with those.

ALLERGY BASICS

ALLERGY AND INTOLERANCE

Let's get some basic terminology out of the way. Two words you're going to hear a lot in this chapter are *allergy* and *intolerance*. Both describe symptoms that happen when you feed a baby. *Allergy is used when symptoms are caused by an immune reaction.* So when the immune system "sees" milk protein, for example, and brings in special cells and antibodies to start a fight, that's a true allergic reaction. In a baby, this usually equates to rash, vomiting, or blood and mucus in the poo.

Intolerance, on the other hand, is when a baby is given something and it causes a problem that doesn't involve the immune system. So, for example, a baby gets gas when she eats green beans. In common language, this is when something simply doesn't "agree" with your baby. Another example is lactose intolerance, which is often confused with milk allergy.

As a parent, you'll face lots of intolerance and probably less allergy. But what's important is to understand and recognize allergy when it happens. This is the reaction that needs attention, since it can lead to other problems down the line if it's not intercepted.

ALLERGY RISING

Allergy is on the rise in developed countries like the United States. Skin, respiratory (asthma), and food allergy have shown a huge jump over the past twenty years. The reason for this bump isn't clear, although one theory is that, as a culture, we've become preoccupied with cleanliness—and the cleaner we've become, the less experienced our children's immune systems have become. As we saw in Chapter 2, this connection between allergy and cleanliness has been called the *hygiene hypothesis*. We'll dive further into that idea in a bit.

ALLERGY—IT'S ALL IN THE FAMILY

Perhaps more important than your baby's exposure to dirt and barnyard animals are the genes she's endowed with. While there are a lot of factors to consider, genetics are important when it comes to allergy. It turns out that having a family history of allergy raises the risk of a baby having allergy considerably. If *both parents* have a history of allergy (that means both had eczema, asthma, and/or food allergies), the risk of their baby having issues is about 40 to 80 percent. If *one parent* carries a history of allergy, the risk is 20 to 40 percent. If you're virginal parents with no history, the risk of your baby developing food allergies is about 5 percent.

PARENTS MAKE MISERABLE ALLERGISTS

The problem with this rise in allergy is that every stool-gazing parent in the free world thinks that their baby is having a reaction to food. If poo changes color or a baby farts in the wrong direction, parents beat a path to their pediatrician demanding an allergy intervention. But the research shows that the majority of suspected food reactions reported by parents aren't allergy. Some 40 percent of people report having a food allergy, but only some 1 to 5 percent actually do. I'm not saying that parents are crazy, but they're definitely hyperobservant.

This is both good and bad. It's good because parental concern keeps babies safe. It's bad because too much worry leads to testing and roaming around the countryside looking for answers to problems that don't exist.

My hope is that this chapter will help stop the madness and allow you to try to stick to the facts.

MILK PROTEIN ALLERGY

When it comes to allergy and your baby, we spend most of our time thinking about and acting on milk allergy. Milk protein found in both breast milk and infant formula account for the majority of food allergies that we see in babies. There are other culprits like soy protein, but milk covers most of the map when it comes to the allergic baby. As it turns out, about 3 to 5 percent of all babies will show some signs of milk protein allergy. And in these babies, most of the signs of protein allergy are on the inside of the body.

While this idea of allergy on the insides makes me a busy guy, it's not very complicated and it's something most parents can grasp if they are given the right information.

ALLERGY AND MAMA'S MILK

Timeless urban legends tell us that babies can't react to their mama's milk. But that's the thing about urban legends—they're not usually true. Ultimately, it all depends on what the mama's eating.

Protein from your diet can get through the breast and into your baby to create a reaction. In fact, babies commonly react to the proteins ingested by breast-feeding moms. But if you're a mom and you're working your tail off to feed your baby with breast milk, I want to make it really clear that your baby is reacting to proteins *in your milk,* not to you.

Your baby can't be allergic to you. That happens when they turn fourteen.

HOW MILK ALLERGY IN A BABY IS UNLIKE THAT KID DOWN THE STREET WITH PEANUT ALLERGY

Food allergy strikes fear into the hearts of hovering parents. The good news is that the allergy that we see in baby guts is different from the kind of reaction typically seen with peanuts. Peanut allergies tend to be *systemic.* In other words, they involve the throat, lungs, and other vital organs that keep us alive. This kind of allergic reaction tends to move pretty quickly. It's scary stuff, for sure.

But the milk allergy that we see in the baby gut is a kind of *slow allergy.* It sometimes takes hours or days to develop, and it typically doesn't involve vital organs like the breathing tube. In this type of allergy, the immune system first "sees" a substance when that substance touches the lining of the intestine. If the baby body sees that substance as foreign, then it sends in white blood cells to react. This "calling in the troops" takes some time to happen.

The challenge here with identifying this kind of slow allergy is that food reactions in babies can be delayed until hours after we've fed them. And this has real impact when you're restricting foods as a breast-feeding mother and then trying to make sense of what's happening in your baby.

POO AS A SIGN OF THE ALLERGY INSIDE

The challenge for me as a poo professional is that the problems I deal with are on the inside. My friends in dermatology have it easy since the skin is right out there for everyone to see. Sure, I have fancy fiber-optic scopes for peeking into stomachs, but we simply can't scope every baby.

So instead we have to look for patterns and signs. We look at the poo and listen to the baby. Poo (and babies) can tell us a lot if we're willing to listen (and look).

THE BABY WITH MILK ALLERGY: ENTER THE TYPICAL SUSPECT

So what does the typical baby with milk allergy look like? What pattern might point to a diagnosis of allergy?

Let's profile the typical allergic suspect.

AGE: FOUR TO SIX WEEKS

Protein allergy normally kicks in after about a month of life, as it takes some time to build. Like the reaction you might have to the metal of a piece of jewelry, the reaction doesn't show up the minute you slip on the offending ring. It takes time for those allergy cells to find their way in and make your skin red. And until those cells show up, you're not going to see much.

BLOOD IN THE POO

Many babies with milk allergy have blood in their poo. Usually it's bright red and appears in stringy streaks. It may come and go, but there can be scary amounts of it at times. Sometimes, though, the blood in the poo is minuscule enough that it can only be seen with special cards for testing blood (see Chapter 7). Typically, there isn't enough blood loss to make babies sick.

STRINGY MUCUS

Along with blood, you'll likely see slimy mucus in the poo. Remember that mucus is something normally made by the colon. It greases the wheels (so to speak) and helps poo move along. But when the colon's unhappy, it makes more mucus. And so your baby's diapers might be heavy with the slimy stuff. Opening the folded diaper of a milk allergic baby will often show the telltale "bridging mucus" sign, where the strings of slime reach from side to side.

DIARRHEA

Some babies will have loose-to-runny stools along with their mucus and blood. In some cases, diarrhea can be a bigger issue because it can create problems with weight gain.

FUSSY, COLICKY BEHAVIOR

Given that the lining of the intestine is inflamed and generally unhappy, the allergic baby in turn is unhappy. She may just be difficult to settle, or she may scream all day long. Some studies show that a significant number of babies labeled with "colic" may be suffering from milk allergy. And if your baby has milk protein allergy, shushing noises and rocking won't make it go away.

THE SPITS AND VOMITS

Keep in mind that the "reaction" between the body and the milk protein can happen anywhere inside a baby, from way up in the swallowing tube to all the way at the very end of the large intestine, right where the poo comes out. This means that the allergic baby can look just like the baby with old-fashioned baby reflux. She may spit up or vomit right after eating, or hours after her feed. During feeding she may be fidgety and fussy, arching and pulling back from the breast or bottle.

MAYBE RASH

Rash (sometimes) happens. While every baby book ever written loves to talk about rash in the allergic baby, as someone who deals with this problem every day I can tell you that rash is overrated. In fact, the majority of babies with proven allergy in my clinic have pristine baby skin. Lots of parents will look at baby acne or random imperfections in the skin and think that it's related to their baby's milk.

When rash does happen, it's typically a scaly "eczema" rash that can occur just about anywhere. It feels like dry, rough skin, but it doesn't get better with moisturizer. Usually it pops up in small, patchy areas the size of a dime, but it can cover a baby's entire body in some cases.

OVERRATED BREATHING PROBLEMS

Breathing problems like wheezing are unusual in milk allergy. Most of what's seen in the allergic baby is in the gut and sometimes on the skin. Allergy can eventually continue its march to involve the lungs, with asthma and wheezing, but that typically won't happen until later in infancy or into toddlerhood.

DISRUPTED SLEEP

While there are a lot of reasons why a baby won't sleep, add milk allergy to the list as well. Studies show that milk protein allergy in babies leads to disrupted sleep.

> ## ALLERGY DOESN'T MAGICALLY APPEAR AT 8 MONTHS
>
> While your baby's allergy could have been mild or under the radar before the middle of her first year, it's pretty unusual that it first appears at that point. If your baby shows allergic signs late in the first year, it may be something different and should be investigated carefully.

SO HOW DO YOU REALLY KNOW IF YOUR BABY'S ALLERGIC?

If you look at the laundry list of allergy signs and symptoms that I've laid out, you may think it's fairly nonspecific. And you're absolutely right. Allergy or no allergy, babies scream and pass mucus in their stool sometimes. And every mother knows that rashes can come and go in babies for all kinds of reasons.

In most cases, the allergy diagnosis is what's called a *clinical diagnosis*. This means that we look at a baby's signs and symptoms, and if they seem to fit allergy, we make the diagnosis. Or put another way, if it walks like a duck and quacks like a duck, it's probably a duck.

Of course, not all ducks look alike. And some ducks don't quack. So diagnosing allergy in a baby can be tricky at times.

Given that most of the problems we see in the milk allergic baby happen on the inside, we can actually tell a lot from peeking in. Using supertiny fiber-optic endoscopes, we can see inside the stomach and colon of potentially reacting babies. Small samples of tissue will usually show allergic cells and clinch the diagnosis.

But the reality is that we can't just stick a scope in a baby whenever we're feeling curious. I'm frequently curious, but that's not a good enough reason. Using a scope is expensive, it has some risk, insurance companies definitely don't like it, it makes young parents crazy nervous, and in many cases it doesn't change things very much. So a scope in the bum for the allergic baby should be a rarity.

Most pediatric tummy docs only turn to a scope when an allergic baby is sick and a firm diagnosis absolutely needs to be made. And if it seems as if your gastroenterologist has a quick hand, you might want to seek a second opinion. Usually we try some other things out before looking with a scope.

But what about more tests? After all, if we can put a supercomputer in our pockets and a man on the moon, surely there must be some other kind of test that can tell us if a baby is allergic . . . (spoiler alert: there isn't). While a food challenge (when you offer a food to see if there's a reaction) is the closest thing to the best test for food allergy, conducting food challenges can be a significant operation requiring serious expertise. Furthermore, it may not be necessary for most babies.

ALLERGY TESTS AND OTHER FANTASIES

As demanding patients and parents of the twenty-first century, we're getting used to the fact that there's a urine dipstick test or

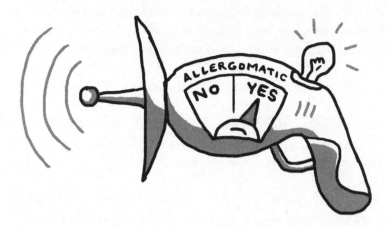

a scan for just about everything. So it's hard to face the fact that there really isn't a reliable, easy-to-conduct test for milk allergy in babies.

There is a blood test that checks for immunoglobulin E (IgE) antibodies to certain things in a child's diet (antibodies are the great big proteins made by the immune system that float around our blood looking for foreign things). The problem is that having antibodies to a protein doesn't mean that you are going to react. For example, I have a handful of antibodies to some common things that I eat every day. The presence of these antibodies doesn't mean that I will react to those foods.

To complicate matters, young babies often carry mom's antibodies. For the first few months, babies carry around what mom gave them in the womb until they start making their own. This makes testing babies a little tricky.

So while there are some exceptions, "allergy testing" babies is problematic.

Skin tests are a little bit more sensitive when it comes to helping us understand what's happening in a youngster, but we can typically only do those once a child hits two or three years of age. Skin testing can be performed in babies to see if allergy is a possibility. If it's negative, allergy is not a concern but intolerance may still be causing symptoms.

When it comes to the allergic baby, ultimately we're dependent on stethoscope-wearing humans who have experience teasing out patterns. What happens with a baby while taking a food verses while avoiding a food is the best way to tell if an allergy is present without relying on fancy, invasive tests.

EOSINOPHILS AND OTHER SUPERSECRET CLUES TO ALLERGY

Actually, we sometimes see things in the blood that can hint of allergy. Babies may have an elevation in *eosinophils,* a type of white blood cell associated with allergy and asthma. We can also see the rise in the IgE antibody. Blood platelets are often elevated as well. So there are a few simple clues to allergy that sometimes can be seen on routine blood testing.

FIXING YOUR BABY'S ALLERGY

OKAY, SO LET's say you've got the screaming, bleeding, mucousy baby with a little bit of eczema who we suspect is reacting to your milk. What can you expect your doctor to do? Or, in this age of empowered patients and parents, what can *you* do?

While you may think you need a doctor to make this diagnosis, how I figure this out is not usually much different from what I've told you here. In fact, after four years of medical school, three years of pediatric residency, three years of pediatric gastroenterology and nutrition fellowship, and twenty years of experience, much of it still comes down to recognizing patterns.

So while you should of course see your doctor in this situation, there's still a lot you can do to help. Because the takeaway is this: how you treat your baby's allergy depends on how you fill your baby's tummy.

TREATING THE BREAST-FED BABY FOR ALLERGY

Understanding the issues in the allergic breast-fed baby are key because too often decisions are made impulsively or without the right information.

If you're breast-feeding, the truth is that small bits of protein from the food you eat will make their way into your milk. And it's these proteins that are creating the problem in your allergic baby. Your pediatrician or allergist may choose to measure blood IgE levels against certain foods. This may help narrow down potential culprits in your diet. Until then, here's what you can do.

CUT MILK AND SOY

Start by tightly restricting milk and soy protein (not soy oil or soy lecithin) in your own diet. This restriction alone is going to fix the majority of babies for mamas reading this book.

SIT AND WAIT

This is the hard part, but it's going to take a couple of days for your milk to clear. Then it's going to take a couple of weeks for your baby's bowel to heal. In the meantime, expect your baby to continue to fuss and show streaks of blood in the diaper. Remember that even if you had changed to a hypoallergenic formula right away instead of restricting milk and soy protein from your diet, the improvement likely wouldn't have been faster. The simple fact is that it takes time for the inflamed baby tummy to heal. There's not a lot that can be done in the meantime.

DON'T PUMP AND DUMP

Many mothers are advised to pump their milk and dump it down the drain while they're waiting for their breast milk to clear. Although this may be standard practice for a lot of pediatricians, it usually isn't necessary. The impact of a little extra protein exposure over a couple of days is offset by the value of all the other good stuff found in your breast milk.

DON'T BE A WEENIE

The most important thing to keep in mind about allergy in the breast-fed baby is that most babies can continue to breast-feed. Many of the babies I see who have been taken off breast milk for allergy have been switched to hypoallergenic formula too early. Often this is done by doctors who don't know any better or who can't stand to tell a mother the hard fact that she's gotta wait. I treat a lot of breast-fed babies with allergic disease and it's infrequent that I ever discontinue breast milk.

WHEN TO MOVE BEYOND YOUR OWN MILK RESTRICTION

So what do you do if you're three weeks in to your own milk and soy restriction and your baby's symptoms of allergy are unchanged? As it turns out, other proteins in your milk can give your baby fits or mucousy poo. In this case, you can usually make the move to cut eggs and nuts, a commonly implicated pair of foods that cause baby allergy. Then you need to wait again, and let your breast milk, and your baby, clear.

BEWARE THE SCORCHED EARTH APPROACH

The scorched earth approach to allergy is when you consider cutting nearly everything (for example, dairy, soy, eggs, nuts, and wheat) from your diet on the day your baby begins having allergy symptoms. This may seem like a good idea, but it's usually not necessary, it's superhard to sustain over the first few months of life, and it puts you at risk of quitting breast-feeding. And while extensive restrictions are unlikely to impact the quality of the breast milk that you produce, the greater risk may be to your own health.

I know you love your baby, but you've got to look after yourself as well (and this little piece of advice will apply for the next eighteen years).

TREATING THE BOTTLE-FED BABY FOR ALLERGY

If you're bottle-feeding with a standard infant formula and your baby shows the signs and symptoms of milk protein allergy, here's what you should do.

SWITCH TO A HYPOALLERGENIC FORMULA

The best thing to do for the allergic baby is to feed her what's called an *extensively hydrolyzed protein formula*. For simplicity's sake, I'll call this a standard hypoallergenic formula.

STANDARD FORMULA

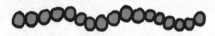

(PROTEIN IS INTACT)

HYPOALLERGENIC FORMULA

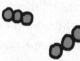

(PROTEIN IS PARTIALLY BROKEN DOWN)

SUPER-DUPER HYPOALLERGENIC FORMULA

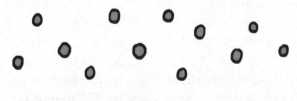

(PROTEIN IS TOTALLY BROKEN DOWN)

It's essentially a formula made with protein that's been sliced and diced so that your baby's immune system doesn't see it as a problem, and it's the first-line treatment for the non-breast-fed baby. The formulas that fit in this category are **Nutramigen, Alimentum**, and **Extensive HA**. You can find them in the grocery store on the Great Wall of Formula.

As mentioned in Chapter 3, hypoallergenic formulas tend to taste like roadkill. If your baby's smart, she'll recognize pretty quickly that this stuff tastes horrible. In fact, she may refuse to drink it at first, but hang in there. Playing hardball will usually work, but for the holdouts we have had luck flavoring a four-to-six-ounce bottle of hypoallergenic formula with two drops of vanilla extract. You can also slowly introduce the formula by mixing a small amount of the hypoallergenic formula into your breast milk (i.e., in a 1:8 ratio) and increase it each day until she's drinking all formula. This will allow your baby's taste buds to adjust. For more on this, see Sweetening Formula on page 258.

SIT AND WAIT

Remember that it takes time for the tummy to heal when you remove the protein that's causing your baby's insides to get irritated and red. The inflammatory cells that are causing the cramping, mucus, misery, and bleeding won't disappear overnight. Once these cells realize that there's no longer something there to react to, they'll simply go about their business in the body looking for other foreign elements.

While you may begin to see some improvement within a few days, it may take up to three weeks for things to really begin to clear. Be patient.

PERFECT POO IS THE ENEMY OF GOOD POO

Here's a hard reality: not every baby with milk protein allergy is going to completely clear with hypoallergenic formula. But if they're considerably improved, they're happier, and their bleeding has decreased significantly, we usually don't recommend doing anything else. In other words, if a baby has occasional streaks of blood in the poo but is happy and healthy otherwise, we usually let that baby continue rollin' with their hypoallergenic formula.

A small amount of irritation in a healthy baby isn't an issue since milk allergy in infancy is typically a short-lived problem. And the hassle of moving to the next category of super-duper hypoallergenic formulas is a bigger deal. Just don't expect perfection in your allergic baby's number two.

SOME BABIES WON'T GET BETTER

About 80 percent of babies will improve on standard hypoallergenic formula. But if you do the math, that means that there will still be 20 percent of babies who continue to react to even those small, diced-up chunks of protein. If a baby continues to have significant tummy symptoms that don't improve, we treat her with a class of super-duper hypoallergenic formulas called *amino-acid-based formula* (more on this next).

SWEETENING FORMULA

If you've never thought about sweetening your baby's hypoallergenic formula, you've obviously never tasted it. Despite its roadkill taste, we flavor hypoallergenic milks only as a last resort. I usually encourage families to play hardball first, and typically the babies come around. Two drops of vanilla extract will sometimes do the trick; occasionally we use a half packet of artificial sweetener (like NutraSweet) when a sick baby desperately needs the milk.

Ultimately, though, your baby's palate is not re-fined enough to require sugar. And excessive sugar can lead to slow intestinal motility, create diarrhea, and promote tooth decay. If your baby has a prob-lem feeding that's bad enough to consider flavoring, get it checked out with your pediatrician first.

SUPER-DUPER FANCY HYPOALLERGENIC FORMULAS AND WHY YOUR BABY MIGHT OR MIGHT NOT NEED THEM

Most babies get better on a standard hypoallergenic formula, but some babies continue to show significant symptoms of gut allergy even after two to three weeks of this formula.

In these cases, we turn to the amino-acid-based formulas men-tioned above. These formulas don't contain any intact protein that the immune system can recognize; instead, they contain amino ac-ids, which are the building blocks of protein. The formulas in this category are **Neocate**, **Elecare**, **PurAmino**, and **Alfamino**.

Amino-acid-based formulas are saved for the sickest babies. They're expensive, they often need to be special ordered, they taste horrible, they smell, and they'll make your baby's poo a creepy ev-ergreen color. If you need them, fine. If you don't, they're best left for a sicker baby.

Perhaps the biggest miscalculation made with the allergic baby is moving to an amino-acid-based formula when either a standard hypoallergenic formula hasn't been given enough time or when a baby really isn't that sick. When waiting, parents often get impatient and put pressure on their pediatricians to pull the trigger on the big guns. Hang in there and stay strong.

So who's sick enough for an amino-acid-based formula? Certainly babies who continue to show allergic symptoms of bleeding, diarrhea, marked irritability, allergy rash, or poor weight despite two to three weeks of extensively hydrolyzed formula use. Sometimes when a baby looks frail and sick from presumed allergy, a number two expert will move straight to an amino-acid-based formula rather than waiting for an extensively hydrolyzed milk to kick in.

SOY: NOT A SOLUTION FOR ALLERGY

About 50 percent of children who are allergic to milk protein will react to soy protein. So unless you're feeling really lucky, soy formula has no place in the treatment of the baby with a milk allergy.

ON CHECKING POO FOR BLOOD

Having treated thousands of babies with allergic disease and dealt with nearly as many pediatricians caring for those babies, I have seen an issue that comes up when evaluating a baby's response to formula: *Should you check for microscopic blood in a baby being treated with a hypoallergenic formula?* I strongly suggest that if a baby's doing well, the presence of microscopic blood shouldn't change what we do or force a change to a super-duper hypoallergenic formula. A little microscopic blood is not an issue given that this is a short-lived problem.

CAN YOU SWITCH FORMULAS YOURSELF, WITHOUT YOUR DOCTOR'S PERMISSION?

Yes, but this depends on the relationship you have with your pediatrician. If you're afraid of him or her, you may feel that this is something you can't do. Though of course, if you've got that kind of fear-based relationship with your child's doctor, I'd suggest that you adjust your perspective as an empowered parent and/or look for another doctor. I'd also suggest that, based on what you've read here in *Number Two*, if you have a baby sick enough to need an amino-acid-based formula, you should be looking for expert help before trying to manage things on your own.

Still, don't fall into the trap of formula roulette. Yes, it's a free country, but that doesn't mean that it makes sense to change formulas more often than you change diapers. For many parents, milk is the single variable in their baby's world that they can control, so they take their chances with formula roulette. And usually it's to fix something that they think is happening inside of their baby. But the only formula change that's going to result in a real difference is the switch made to treat allergy.

Remember that a lot of infant feeding is voodoo promulgated by formula manufacturers preying on the tired and frustrated.

Where you least expect it | Places where you can find milk protein

High-protein flour	Butter and Margarine	Chocolate
Nondairy creamer	Brown sugar flavoring	Deli meats
Cottage cheese	Custard	Curd
Ghee (clarified butter)	Nougat	Caramel flavoring
Saltines	Batter-dipped veggies	Fast food french fries

THE GREAT LACTOSE-FREE CONSPIRACY

The biggest infant-feeding scam that you may get pulled into is the treatment of lactose intolerance. Let's start with a little basic digestive physiology. Grab a chair and stick with me because if you don't understand this, you'll never understand why you're getting scammed.

Lactose is the basic sugar found in milk. After milk is swallowed, it goes through the stomach and into the small intestine. Lactose, the milk sugar, is broken down and absorbed by an enzyme called lactase, which is found on the lining of the small intestine. The by-products of this breakdown, glucose and galactose, are absorbed and used for energy and growth in our bodies.

Are you with me so far?

Every baby has lactase. But at some point during the school-age years or young adulthood, some people stop making lactase, or stop making it at 100 percent (some people will make 50 percent of their enzyme, for example). This happens because of a genetic switch that decides that lactase isn't needed anymore.

Stay with me.

If a person stops making the lactase enzyme, lactose will not be absorbed in the small intestine as it's supposed to. And in that case, the lactose in our food keeps moving downstream until it hits the colon and encounters those hundred trillion bacteria we talked about in Chapter 3. Now, bacteria love sugar. So they have a big party there in the colon and eat the lactose. As a by-product of this bacterial digestion (in a process called fermentation), stinky gas is produced, in addition to other stuff that gives you diarrhea, cramps, and a growly, grumbly stomach.

We call this lactose intolerance. This is an *intolerance*. It is not an allergy. The symptoms arise from the failure of the intestinal tract to process and absorb milk sugar. It has nothing to do with the immune system and there is no reaction.

BABIES AND LACTOSE INTOLERANCE

So where does your baby fit into this? Actually, she doesn't. Or she can't.

Hang on, we're almost there.

In the history of modern medicine, only a handful of babies have been born without the ability to make lactase. These are rare, historical cases that get published in fancy, highfalutin journals. Unless you personally gave birth to one of the half dozen or so affected, your baby will not have an issue with lactose and, consequently, her problems will never be "fixed" by lactose-free formula.

But, you may argue, there are lactose-free formula options on the Great Wall of Formula. You are correct. This is a deliberate attempt by formula manufacturers to bamboozle you and steal your money. Young, impressionable, stool-gazing parents who have not read *Looking Out for Number Two* may believe that their gassy baby is "allergic to lactose." But as I've explained, one can't be allergic to lactose, and a baby born with an absence of lactase is a historical event.

And when a baby has an immune reaction to milk protein (that's an allergy), it has nothing to do with milk sugar.

Capisce?

So if you've got some crazy person tellin' you that your baby has lactose intolerance, then send them a copy of this book. More important, if you have a pediatrician who tells you that your baby needs lactose-free formula for allergy, it's time to find another pediatrician.

TEMPORARY LACTOSE INTOLERANCE
Babies can become *temporarily* intolerant of lactose when they're recovering from a severe stomach virus.

The lining of the intestine can lose its lactase while the virus runs rampant, but it comes back after a few days when the bowel heals. Research studies are mixed about whether the removal of lactose during this short time makes a difference.

WHY GOAT'S MILK IS ONLY FOR FOUR-LEGGED KIDS

If you ask enough people about unhappy or allergic babies, goat's milk as a remedy will eventually come up. Let's save you some time and heartache here and just say that this is advice that you can leave on the Internet or wherever you got it.

Goat's milk is made for goats and not for (human) kids.

Used for years as a cure-all for fussy babies, goat's milk was considered easier for babies to digest. Although it does form a softer curd in the stomach (the curd is the cheesy stuff you see in a baby's spit-up), it's not an appropriate source of nutrition for babies because of its nutrient balance and high level of protein.

Goat's milk is deficient in vitamins B and C, folate, and iron. It contains levels of sodium, potassium, and protein that are way too high for a baby's kidneys. While in the short term goat's milk won't create a problem, its concentration of minerals can be life-threatening should a baby continue to drink it when sick or dehydrated.

This may appear to be goat discrimination, but the same also applies to the sacred cow. Both goat's milk *and* cow's milk are verboten for babies and should be withheld under a year of age. Despite its popularity with past generations, say no to goat's milk or cow's milk out of the carton unless your baby is twelve months or older (or happens to be a goat or a cow).

THE NATURAL HISTORY OF THE MILK ALLERGIC BABY

What happens to the baby with milk allergy as she grows older?

Not much, really. Because milk allergy in babies isn't forever. In fact, by the time most milk allergic babies hit seven to nine months of age, they can transition back to standard infant formula without a problem. Crisis averted. Problem gone.

There are, however, a few things to keep in mind when bringing your baby back into the world of milk.

THERE'S NO LOGIC TO GRADUAL TRANSITIONS

Some parents are advised to mix their hypoallergenic formula with regular formula to gradually introduce milk protein to their baby: 50:50, then 60:40, followed by 70:30. The reality is that when the allergic reactivity that we see in babies is gone, it's gone. Gradual transitions serve no role in helping your baby. This kind of hocus-pocus won't prevent your baby from reacting and it certainly won't allow her to "get used to it." In fact, it may even make it difficult to see if your baby is truly experiencing ongoing allergy to milk. I recommend a straight switch to standard formula after eight months if a child is otherwise well.

IF STANDARD FORMULA IS TOLERATED, A BABY CAN ADVANCE ON TO WHOLE MILK AT A YEAR

Should all go well with exposure to standard infant formula, it's okay to transition to milk out of the carton at a year. If your baby does well with this, ice cream on her first birthday is fine. Your mileage may vary.

SOME BABIES WILL CONTINUE TO REACT

A small number of babies will continue to react to milk protein even at their first birthday. The percentage of babies that do this is very small, so the odds are in your favor that this won't be the case. If allergy continues, though, you will typically see symptoms similar to the ones your baby had early in life. Fussiness, vomiting, diarrhea or increased poo, and disrupted sleep are the biggest signs that allergic inflammation may be making a comeback. It may take two to four days to see a problem.

WHOLE MILK IS OVERRATED

A lot of the anxiety surrounding milk allergy in babies centers on the concern over starting whole milk around a year. But for many babies after a year of age, milk isn't necessary. We've all been brainwashed to believe that milk is a critical part of every child's diet. But the truth is that it's nothing more than a vehicle for calories, protein, and calcium. These three nutritional components are important, don't get me wrong. But many toddlers get all the nutrition they need through their diet.

That being said, milk may play a helpful role in maintaining a healthy diet for the dangerously picky toddler.

SOLID FOOD AND THE ALLERGIC BABY

FEEDING SOLIDS TO YOUR MILK ALLERGIC BABY

While special milk may work to make your screaming bundle of allergic misery happy, the day will come when you have to start your baby on solid food. This usually makes parents very nervous because they don't want a repeat performance of what they experienced in the first month or two of their baby's life.

As it turns out, most of the worry isn't backed up with real risk. Babies with milk allergy typically advance on baby food just like every other baby at six months of age. The first foods that we feed babies don't contain proteins that typically cause allergy, so the introduction of solids rarely creates problems for the majority of milk allergic babies.

CAN YOU PREVENT ALLERGY TO BEGIN WITH?

FEAR OVER ALLERGY, especially when there is a family history, often starts well before a baby is born. A lot of families have experience with an allergic baby or know that they carry a strong family history of allergy. Parents often want to know what they can do early on to minimize their baby's risk, and they frequently ask me what, if anything, they should feed their baby to *prevent* allergy. Let's take a closer look.

FOOD CHOICES DURING PREGNANCY | OR WHY ICE CREAM AND PICKLES ARE STILL OKAY

The most recent studies show that the restriction of cow's milk and eggs during pregnancy doesn't influence a baby's risk of developing allergies later. The studies on how peanut popping while pregnant affects the later risk of peanut allergy are unclear and so recommendations in either direction can't be made. Thus far, there's little evidence to show that what you eat or don't eat during pregnancy can help reduce the initial risk of allergy.

Regarding lactation, no conclusive evidence exists to support the idea that restrictions while breast-feeding will impact your baby's risk for later allergy. Keep in mind that if your baby *already shows signs of allergy,* restriction will be necessary, as we discussed earlier in the chapter.

CHOOSING JUST THE RIGHT MILK TO MINIMIZE RISK

As it turns out, you may be able to do a couple of things to minimize allergy risk.

The first and best way to minimize risk of allergy in your baby is to breast-feed. Breast milk decreases the odds of a baby developing milk allergy, eczema, and wheezing.

In fact, even the simple exposure to cow's milk (like that found in infant formula) *during the first week of life* increases the odds of developing allergy over fourfold. Cow's milk protein exposure *during the first several months of life* increases allergy risk threefold over babies fed exclusively with human milk. Those are scary stats.

But the reality is that not every mother can breast-feed. So when it comes to formula-fed babies, what can you do instead?

As it turns out, you can feed your baby certain kinds of milk protein that will decrease their odds of developing food allergy.

Some studies show that babies with a hereditary risk for allergy (parental allergy that was either patient reported or physician diagnosed) who are fed *partially digested milk protein* are at lower risk of developing food allergies during childhood.

In the German Infant Nutrition Initiative (GINI) study, babies were fed different kinds of milk during infancy and then were followed for a decade to see how their risk for allergy measured up. Babies fed partially digested milk proteins had a lower risk of developing allergic symptoms over those next ten years. It seems that when proteins are partially broken down, the immune system is less likely to attack the non-broken-down versions of these proteins and others later on. And thus the simple adjustment of the kind of proteins given to a baby can impact their allergy risk.

If you turn back to Chapter 4 on formulas, you'll remember that there are different kinds of formulas based on the kinds of proteins that they contain. The formulas that are made up of partially digested proteins are Nutramigen, Alimentum, Extensive HA, and Good Start.

This impact of infant feeding on the development of allergy is so compelling that the American Association of Allergy Asthma and Immunology released recommendations in 2014 suggesting that any child from a family with a history of allergy should be given a formula with partially hydrolyzed milk protein. So if you have a family history of food allergy, you can't breast-feed, and you want to minimize risk in your baby, consider using a formula with partially digested proteins. But a 2016 review article (a study of studies) published in the British Medical Journal explored this protein-allergy connection and refuted the claim that partially digested protein can prevent allergy. Stay tuned, as the story is evolving.

If this connection between cow's-milk exposure in infancy and the ultimate development of allergy is proven to be correct, then it's possible that by the time you have grandchildren, we won't be using the regular infant formulas available today.

STARTING SOLIDS AND THE RISK OF ALLERGY IN YOUR BABY

Another widely discussed allergy hack is the practice of delaying solids to avoid allergy. On a certain level this seems to make sense, as the idea is to allow the immune system to grow up a bit. But this timeless urban legend also supports my idea that parents make terrible allergists.

As it turns out, there is no consistent evidence that withholding solids beyond four to six months does anything to prevent allergy in your baby. In fact, the contrary may even be true: the delayed introduction of solids may raise the risk of eczema or food allergy. As discussed earlier in this chapter and in Chapter 3, you should start your baby on a sequence of solids beginning around six months of age or a little earlier. There are many good reasons for getting your baby out of the gate with a bowl and spoon by this age, even beyond allergy.

Regarding allergenic foods like nuts and eggs, evidence supports the idea that these can be given during the first year after a few basic foods have been started (cereal and veggies). In fact, recent studies support the idea that the introduction of eggs during the first year may actually help *reduce* the risk of egg allergy later. Related studies have shown that peanut allergy can actually be *prevented* by the introduction of peanut into an infant's diet between four and eleven months of age.

However, if your family has a strong history of allergy or your baby has already established allergy or eczema, consult an allergist or your pediatrician.

CAN YOU FEED (OR NOT FEED) TO PREVENT CELIAC DISEASE?

If poo is the new parental preoccupation, gluten is not far behind it. Let's turn to celiac disease and what we can and shouldn't do when it comes to gluten and our babies.

WHAT IS CELIAC DISEASE?

Celiac disease is a condition where gluten, a protein found in wheat, reacts with the lining of the intestine, leading to damage. This injury to the lining of the intestine puts the gut at risk of not doing its job of absorbing nutrients and energy. In children, gluten-induced injury results in malabsorption, leading to diarrhea, abdominal pain, and failure to grow properly.

Studies have shown that as doctors we too often miss the diagnosis of celiac disease. But because of a growing awareness (or obsession) with gluten-related issues, there has been a lot of conspiratorial thinking about gluten. So much thinking, in fact, that gluten has been implicated in nearly every childhood ailment ever identified. If you were to believe most parenting circles, you'd think that gluten restriction offers your child the chance to avoid digestive self-destruction, irrespective of what may be wrong.

If you can find your way around my disbelief, you'll hopefully understand that concern over gluten and its relationship to an endless list of conditions is overstated. If your child suffers from celiac disease, that's one thing. Otherwise, gluten restriction should have no place on your parental radar.

CAN YOU CONTROL YOUR BABY'S CELIAC RISK BY HOLDING THE GLUTEN?

For families at risk for celiac disease or those who've had a close encounter with celiac disease, it's reasonable to ask about the timing of gluten introduction in their baby as a means of preventing celiac disease.

So what's the scoop? According to the latest recommendations from the European Society of Pediatric Gastroenterology, Hepatology & Nutrition (ESPGHAN), gluten can be introduced to your baby's diet at any point between four and twelve months. A recent study in the *New England Journal of Medicine* found that neither breast-feeding nor the delay of gluten introduction to at-risk babies (those with an affected first degree family member and the high-risk celiac gene) changed the ultimate risk of developing celiac disease. Bottom line: if it's in your genes, there's not a lot you can do.

Since recommendations have fluctuated from year to year, what we understand about gluten introduction in babies and the ultimate risk of celiac disease may be a moving target. Perhaps the future will bring a clearer answer or solution. Until then, let them eat bread.

FARTS, COLIC, AND OTHER THINGS THAT MAKE NOISE

Look out for number one and try not to step in number two.
—RODNEY DANGERFIELD

UNDERSTANDING BABY FARTS

NOT EVERYTHING THAT comes out of a baby can be scooped up, wiped off, or thrown away. There are some intangibles that still make themselves known by sound or smell. To start, let's talk gas.

UNDERSTANDING YOUR PRECIOUS LITTLE GASBAG

When it comes to the stuff that comes out of babies, gas is one thing that can make every parent crazy.

Here's why:

1. It comes out of nowhere.

2. It makes babies cry.

3. We can't control it.

4. It smells.

I can come up with others, but the preceding are probably reasons enough to make baby farts (or the inability to fart) one of parenting's key preoccupations.

So where does gas come from and what can you do about it? When I read parenting literature on baby farts (which is how I spend a lot of my time these days), I'm always surprised that few ever approach the core issue of where gas originates. There's no shortage of folksy remedies, but nothing addresses what makes gas come from your cherub's behind.

Stick with me, and I'll help you do the seemingly impossible: get a handle on the baby fart.

START WITH THE UNDERSTANDING THAT BABIES ARE GAS MACHINES

So much of my work as a pediatric gastroenterologist is managing expectations. And one thing that you've got to expect from your baby is gas. It's just what they do. They eat air and make air as part of their new, emerging fourth trimester physiology. Do yourself a favor and accept that gas is part of your baby's life, and then work from there.

FART PHYSICS 101: GAS COMES FROM ONLY TWO PLACES

Before I went to medical school I had to take physics. Physics is

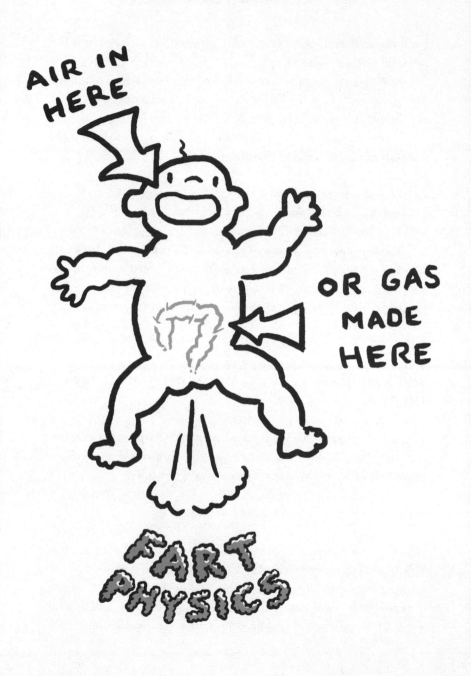

a scientific discipline covering the universal laws that govern the physical world around us.

As it turns out, gas has some universal laws as well. In fact, it's one of the few things that come out of a baby that we can boil down to absolute, unequivocal principles.

I'll cut right to the chase here and tell you that your baby's gas can only come from one of two places:

1. Gas comes from swallowed air.
2. Gas is made by bacteria.

There is no other source of gas in your baby. Period. Let's call this the universal law of baby farts. You won't read about this in the *New England Journal of Medicine* or the *Journal of Pediatrics,* but the nice thing about being a parenting author is that you can create your own laws.

WHEN THINKING ABOUT THE BOTTOM, TAKE IT FROM THE TOP

When facing a gassy baby, the first thing to think about is whether that baby may be sucking air. Air swallowing is the most over-looked problem in fixing gas. Here's what's behind it.

A BUM LATCH

If you're breast-feeding, you should start by looking at your baby's latch. An open-mouth latch with a nice seal is what we're looking for. Squeaking, squawking, and dribbling may be signs that your baby's got a bum latch and she's suckin' and swallowin' wind. If there's any question about this, an evaluation by an experienced lactation consultant can settle the issue and offer solutions if need be.

A BUM NIPPLE

If you're bottle-feeding your baby, think about the nipple. A nipple with a flow that's *too low* will result in a desperately hungry baby who will suck and pull, only to take in air from around the nipple. A nipple with a flow that's *too high* will deliver too much milk, with resulting sputtering, gagging, and air ingestion.

Notice that I didn't say anything about your bottle system. When your baby has a bad connection at the nipple, investing in some cockamamie bottle system with voodoo claims about gas is like rearranging lounge chairs on the deck of the *Titanic*. It's the wrong place to put your energy.

You can change bottle systems, but be sure to put your attention on the nipple and the latch.

POOR POSITIONING

In nearly all respects, babies do better feeding in a semiupright position. This also allows milk to go down and air to come up as much as possible. Although positioning isn't a deal breaker, it's a small thing that can have big results.

If you don't believe me, try drinking from a sports bottle while lying in bed and report back.

PAINFUL SWALLOWING

As we talked about in Chapter 6, if a baby experiences pain when she swallows, she's likely to exhibit what I like to call chaotic feeding. That's the phenomenon where the baby sucks, feels pain, pulls away, and then realizes that she's still hungry. This is not good for you or your baby. If you're breast-feeding, it will ultimately tear the daylights out of your nipples and potentially corrupt your ability to breast-feed. Most important, when a baby breaks her latch or pulls from the bottle, she swallows air. Fixing painful feeding means understanding and addressing the source, and reflux and allergy are a couple of the prime suspects. If you haven't already, check out Chapters 6 and 10 for more information.

SHAKEN FORMULA

When it comes to powdered formula, babies prefer their formula gently stirred, not shaken. I can't count the number of times I've evaluated a terminally gassy baby only to watch mama fill the bottle with powder and water and shake it over her shoulder like some kinda showy bartender making a martini.

James Bond preferred his martinis shaken, not stirred. But your baby's no 007.

Shaken formula is loaded with mini microbubbles that gang up to make megabubbles. If you feel compelled to shake, let it settle before feeding. Otherwise stir gently or use ready-to-feed formula.

THE BIG VICIOUS GASSY CYCLE

Perhaps the biggest source of gas in the screaming baby is the screaming itself. When babies scream for whatever reason, they swallow air. I see this every day in my busy practice: parents fall into the trap of thinking that a baby is suffering from gas when, in fact, they're suffering from something different that causes screaming and air ingestion.

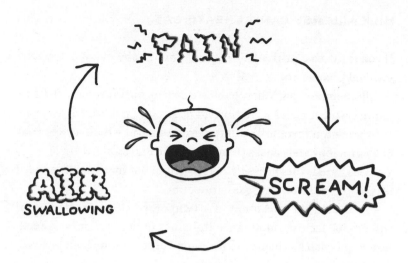

And the more they scream, the more air they swallow, which makes them scream more and leads to the *Big Vicious Gassy Cycle*.

To break the BVGC, you have to get to the root of why a baby may be so dang unhappy. In most cases, this involves going after the king and queen of baby irritability: reflux and allergy. But you should consider constipation and other problems with number two as well. Starvation as a means of controlling reflux is another biggie, because (spoiler alert), hungry babies cry.

LACK OF BURPING

What you can't prevent in terms of swallowing you might be able to catch before it goes beyond the tummy. Don't forget to help your baby make a great, big burp while feeding. Frequent burping represents one of the most basic forms of gas prophylaxis.

MILK ALLERGY CAN'T CREATE GAS

If you think that milk allergy can give your baby gas, you officially flunked Chapter 10.

Remember that when babies react to milk protein, the immune system creates irritation *but no gas is generated*. Instead, the inflammation from milk allergy creates pain, which makes your baby unhappy and causes them to scream and swallow air.

Gas here is the *end result, not the cause*. But that's as close as I'll let you get in the allergy-gas connection.

And with the exception of a temporary situation after viral infections, lactose intolerance in babies effectively doesn't exist. Again, go back to Chapter 10 for more information about milk allergy and lactose intolerance.

Take this to the bank: there are essentially no infant fart problems that can be fixed with a formula change. When it comes to gas, don't be tempted by formula roulette.

GAS CAN BE MADE BELOW

Only after you've considered what's happening above does it make sense to think about what's happening below. So in keeping with our absolute, incontrovertible, universal baby gas laws, if it isn't swallowed, it's made.

This brings us back to the babybiome, one of the most important organs in a baby's body.

THE BABYBIOME EVOLVES WEEK BY WEEK

Remember that your baby's bacterial poo print is in a constant state of evolution. Starting from zero and growing to a mind-blowing one hundred trillion bacteria in the first few days, it doesn't stop there. As dietary fuel for bugs changes during the first year, new materials for the production of gas appear. Throw in antibiotics, exposure to new and wild bugs in day care, and the introduction of exotic baby food, for example, and you can see that gas production becomes part of the babybiome's job.

DIETARY CAUSES OF GAS IN YOUR BABY

As we discussed in Chapter 10, the malabsorption of sugars like lactose can lead to fermentation and gas production by bacteria. But in babies, this is only ever the case after viral infections, and it tends to be short-lived. So don't waste your money on lactose-free formulas.

Remember that when you start solid food, you're fueling your baby's bugs with new kinds of carbohydrates and even fiber that's indigestible. This leads to changes in the biome and changes in the type and volume of gas that your baby makes. So if you've started solids and your baby is extra gassy, make a shift in what you're feeding. Change cereals, drop the fruit that you've just started, or move to a more balanced menu with a complement of cereal, fruit, veggies, and milk.

The sugar found in juices can overrun the gut's capacity to absorb it. So if you've gone beyond two or three ounces of diluted juice per day in your baby of over four months of age, that's one place you may be able to get a leg up on gas.

TWEAK THE BABYBIOME

After a viral infection or the use of antibiotics, the babybiome will undergo a major (but hopefully temporary) shift. Depending upon what population of bugs is obliterated and which ones move in to take over the empty real estate, you could be facing rogue gas makers that scavenge even the smallest remnants of indigestible carbohydrates. As is often the case after antibiotics, a baby's biome fingerprint will migrate back to its set level. But until then, you might face gas that smells different—and there may be more of it.

In this case, the use of a good probiotic will do the trick to restore babybiome basics. I won't spill the beans just yet, but we'll cover probiotics in greater detail in the next chapter.

IT CAN'T GET OUT

While not a common situation, the anatomic bottom problems that lead to the obstruction of poo flow (anal narrowing, incomplete development, etc.) can lead to an overgrowth of nasty bugs. Chronic constipation, continuous straining, and explosive runny mucousy stools may be signs that your pediatrician should investigate via a compulsive medical history and a physical exam that includes the bottom.

COTTON SWAB BEWARE: STICKS AND TRICKS FOR RELEASING GAS

Good parents try things. And they often discover maneuvers that either fix their baby or help them cope with a painful situation. This is usually good, but not always.

Some parents have found that tweaking the bottom with a cotton swab or wiping the anus aggressively with a wet wipe will stimulate elimination or passage of gas. There are even companies marketing sticks or wands specifically designed to tickle the bum.

These are fine for very occasional use in helping gas pass. But just like with pooping, babies have to learn to relax their bottoms in order to release gas. Stimulation is a good short-term solution, but long term it can lead to a baby's inability to do what she needs to do on her own.

POSITIONING FOR THE PERFECT BABY FART | HACKING THE HAUSTRAL TRAP

So much of helping your baby centers around *positioning*. We've seen this theme appear throughout *Looking Out for Number Two* with reflux, burping, and the passage of poo, and it holds true for gas as well.

When we get down to it, the pain your little gasbag experiences comes from small, localized areas of the intestinal tract where large bubbles collect and create painful stretching. In the colon, for example, there are dilated segments called *haustrae* that make the colon look like a string of plump, tasty sausages from the outside. Without getting too deep into it, these dilated segments make perfect areas for gas to hang out and to create havoc for your baby.

So just like burping where we're working to get that big tummy bubble over the lower esophageal sphincter, in the colon we're trying to get gas to move to the next segment of bowel and ultimately free and clear.

Here are a few maneuvers you can try to help move things along:

- **Change the axis.** Move front to back, back to front, or flat to upright. Remember that air goes up, so subtle changes in a baby's position will facilitate the movement of air.
- **Movements.** Beyond creating the right flexed angle, movement in the form of gentle, rhythmic jiggling consolidates smaller air bubbles and helps them move along. The classic

bicycle movement of a baby's legs helps air not only consolidate, but it creates the right position to let air pass from the bottom.

- **Stimulation.** Using two fingers, perform a gentle downward massage on the left side of your baby's belly to stimulate the movement of gas and potentially colonic contractions.

GAS DROPS AND OTHER FORMS OF MODERN WITCHCRAFT

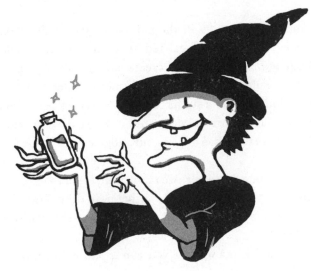

As MUCH AS it pains me, we need to have a discussion about gas drops. Gas drops can be found under any number of names, and those names almost universally make a promise of neonatal bliss. Invariably the word *calm* is used in the name to create the illusion that if you use them, your baby will be calm. *Gripe water* is another common concoction that you'll hear about. While I frequently encounter babies who scream their asses off, I have never seen a baby gripe. If I were the marketing guy at the gas drop company, I'd probably rebrand it as *Scream-your-ass-off water*. If, on the other hand, I were looking for drops to specifically counter the back talk from my twelve-year-old premenarchal daughter, gripe water would seem to offer just the right solution.

Suffice it to say that little of what you may find in gas drops has been proven in clinical studies to do anything to soothe your baby. And as soon as an herb is proven ineffective, another hits the market as part of a never-ending promotional cycle intended to bamboozle you, the frazzled and desperate mama (or papa, or nana).

Although isolated positive results have been reported with the use of fennel extract, chamomile, vervain, licorice, and balm mint, these studies have not been replicated. And some of these products contain sucrose and glucose, which may independently have some effect on making your little bundle of misery more miserable.

SIMETHICONE AND REVERSE LOGIC

The old standby in the battle against gas is simethicone. Simethicone is a compound that's supposed to work by taking small bubbles and making them into big bubbles that are theoretically easier to pass. As the logic goes, it's easier to move a consolidated, well-formed fart than a stream of ill-defined foam.

But given the physiologic mechanics of how gas wreaks colonic havoc in babies, it would make more sense to want the gas to be broken up and not consolidated. Despite the fact that this stuff has been around since the Stone Age, studies show that it effectively does zilch.

Perhaps more important, these controlled studies are supported by the fact that after twenty years of working with such babies, I've yet to see so much as a single baby show improvement with simethicone.

WHY THE BILLION-DOLLAR GAS DROP INDUSTRY WILL NEVER FAIL

Whether gas drops work or not is actually irrelevant. When your baby screams, all logic goes out the window. Here's why you're likely to jump on the gas drop bus.

DON'T JUST STAND THERE, DO SOMETHING

Parents are generally prone to action. And while there is no magic pill, they are led to believe that there just might be. It feels good to do something rather than nothing.

CAN'T HURT, MIGHT HELP

The billion-dollar colic industry is driven by the illogical parental belief that if it can't hurt, it might help. And more important to a parent than any kind of empiric evidence is the fact that of the 567 negative comments on the gas drop forum, one parent actually reported a modicum of relief. This is kind of like playing Powerball and engaging in the fantasy of what it's going to be like to pose for the press when you get that oversized check at lottery headquarters.

DESPERATE PARENTS LOVE THEIR PLACEBOS

Blind studies looking at colic cures (in which parents don't know what the baby's getting) often show very high placebo responses. That means that the parents of babies who got the substance with nothing in it often report dramatic results. As parents, we're very open to suggestion when faced with the stress of a baby in pain. So as long as there's gas and parents looking to release it, there will be a market looking to meet the demand.

THE VAST COLIC CONSPIRACY

LET'S JUMP INTO colic for just a moment. But only for a moment. As you will see after we take a closer look at this scourge of twentieth-century baby rearing, colic may not be all that it's cracked up to be. Or as research is beginning to show, it may represent something new and different. And it may be something you can actually control.

SCREAMING BABIES

There's nothing worse than a screaming baby. Looking after an eight-pound creature is one thing; looking after a screaming, inconsolable eight-pound creature is another thing altogether. When we signed up for a baby, none of us requested this.

I've looked after hundreds, if not thousands of screaming babies. More important, I've looked after twice as many parents desperately coping with their bundles of misery (typically babies have at least two other people impacted by their issues).

Here's why screaming babies are such a problem for new parents:

- We don't know why the screaming is happening.
- We can't control it.
- We don't want our babies to hurt.
- Screaming can drive you to the limits of your sanity.

The stress these little guys put on parents is carried into the exam room, where parents demand answers. And this used to be supereasy for pediatricians, because there was only one diagnosis for babies who fussed: colic. That has changed over the last several years, but as a result, caring for screaming babies is now hard on doctors as well.

A SHORT HISTORY OF COLIC

Not quite a hundred years ago, a bunch of guys got together and decided that when babies cry, it was a definable condition. And since every condition needs scientific-sounding criteria, they deemed that crying lasting three hours a day for at least three days a week that went away at three months of age was to be called colic. And so it was.

The rest is history. And in medicine, it's really hard to shake something that has a name. Doctors like things with names. Especially when they have no idea what's going on.

Pediatricians had it easy once there was a turnkey diagnosis to cover everything that they couldn't begin to understand. They were free from stressed-out mothers looking for answers. With an authoritative nod and a reassuring pat on the back, parents were told to wrap their babies up and take 'em home. It's obviously colic. Let nature take its course.

For doctors, the "discovery of colic" was one of the greatest achievements of the twentieth century—while also its greatest scam. Doctors were absolved of responsibility and parents were left holding the baby. And to this day, we're left with the name—colic as an escape option still remains in play. (Not for me, actually. I don't use the term.)

THE COCKAMAMIE SCIENCE OF COLIC

"Evidence-based" treatments for the dark age diagnosis of colic are centered on the rule of threes (crying for three hours a day at least three days a week in the first three months of age). But

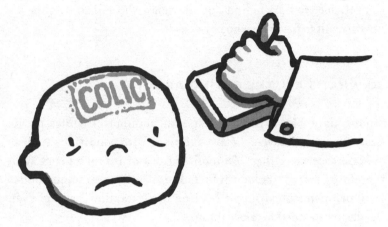

you can't study and measure a problem that was arbitrarily defined to begin with. And colic scientists who perpetuate crying as a disease draw their paychecks from funding bodies that support their colic research. Few studying colic are likely to publicly concede what the rest of medicine knew long ago: that colic is a loosely defined wastebasket diagnosis when we as doctors are short on ideas.

The big problem is this: if your baby cries for two hours and forty-five minutes a day, you're shit out of luck and better look for another diagnosis.

Actually, hold the phone . . . maybe you're not. The "diagnosis" of colic has become bastardized as doctors have individually decided to shape their own harebrained rules and pet theories about crying babies. Everything from a baby's posture to even her response to a vacuum cleaner has been applied in "making the diagnosis." And given the obvious problem with the three-hour rule, ask any pediatrician and they will universally admit that they've abandoned these almost random qualifying criteria.

Colic is the ultimate garbage diagnosis for all seasons. While you will need to work to find a pediatrician who will admit this, it's not difficult to find one who believes it.

SO WHAT'S ALL THE CRYING ABOUT?

Studies have shown that a substantial number of babies previously thought to have colic are suffering with conditions such as allergic disease. Other common sources of infant misery (and therefore crying) include reflux, breast-milk oversupply, lousy latch or mismatched nipple leading to air swallowing, and even the desperate need to take a dump.

Overlying all this are the variable temperaments that we see in different babies, compounded by the variable expectations of their caregivers. And as for the classic crying "witching hour" often referenced in the late afternoon and early evening? This likely represents a pooped-out, fourth trimester brain that has an inability to cope with whatever's making the baby feel off.

In fact, at the end of most days I feel like these babies sound. I've just learned to contain myself (usually).

THE COLIC COTTAGE INDUSTRY

The baby industry loves colic because they want to sell you things. Drops, potions, fragrant skin balms, swings, noisemakers, apps, books, and CDs all offer solutions. In 2007, I bucked the system and published a book called *Colic Solved,* which suggested what all colic capitalists feared: some babies routinely diagnosed with colic may actually be suffering from conditions like allergy and reflux. Those most invested in colic as a cash cow lashed out—and I learned pretty quickly that when you mess with someone's colic business model, you're messin' with their ability to fund their summer house in the Hamptons.

But the good news is that as we've spawned a new generation of pediatricians, awareness of the treatable causes of extreme fussiness has risen. Few babies are wrapped up and sent home without consideration of what could really be going on.

CREATIVE SHUSHING NOISES

In 2002, pediatrician Harvey Karp sold the idea that shushing noises settled babies. He took what doting grandmothers had known for centuries, put it in a book, got coronated by Oprah, and suddenly shushing noises were back in fashion.

To his credit, Karp validated and packaged the concept of soothing noises, which was a really important step. Parents who made a science out of shushing felt empowered by their ability to actually do something. I happen to be a fan of the neutralizing noises promulgated by Karp.

But the fact is that soothing noises work for just about everything that makes babies crazy, from gas to middle ear fluid to a pinkie nail that Grandma clipped too close. I encourage soothing noises and I think you should make them. But I don't encourage overlooking problems that should be considered, diagnosed, and treated.

RETHINKING BABY SCREAMING

Things have changed since the 1950s, when all crying was a single diagnosis. Here's how our understanding of the miraculous baby gut has changed things—or, more specifically, why a catchall diagnosis no longer works.

- The problem of allergy in infancy has grown.
- Infant endoscopic technology has evolved to allow us to identify and understand different kinds of intestinal inflammation.
- Reflux monitoring has developed, and as a result we've learned that even things like positioning in a car seat can set a baby up to scream. And beyond positioning, studies have also shown that about half of all documented reflux events in the pediatric age aren't acid at all, but bile and other digestive juices that create painful symptoms. So even what we understand about reflux has changed very recently.
- The rise of motility as a pediatric specialty has identified the variations and differences in squeezing patterns that change with age and maturity.

Now, there aren't solutions to all these issues, but understanding the root of the problem is a place to start. The point is that there are many reasons babies cry, and we've just begun to scratch the surface.

And just like there isn't only one reason babies cry, there isn't only one diagnosis. I wish it were that simple. It would make my life a whole lot easier.

A WAILING BABY IS NOT A REFLECTION OF YOUR CAPACITY AS A CAREGIVER

Some doctors immediately conclude that irritable babies are a sign that a new mom is having a problem coping. Unfortunately, a variety of degrading terms are attached to the desperate mother advocating for her baby. It's assumed that she's having difficulty adjusting, or that she's too anxious. The inability of a baby to feed or sleep has even been blamed on postpartum depression.

In other words, in the eyes of these providers, it's not their inability to understand your baby, it's your failure to cope with being a new parent. But you need to remember that living with, caring for, and feeding a baby with intestinal disease—or even simple air swallowing—can be incredibly taxing on you and your family. And remember that despite what you're going through, this is not a reflection on you or your ability to be a great mom or dad.

While support for the parents who are experiencing an irritable baby is critical, it's perhaps more critical to have a doctor who is willing to spend more than two minutes looking at a baby. Pediatricians should be willing to spend some time thinking about a baby's problems rather than tattooing a phantom diagnosis on a baby's forehead.

If you're in either of these situations, vote with your feet and find someone who will listen to you and your baby.

THE DYSBIOSIS DIAGNOSIS

As another illustration of just how much things have changed since the 1950s, it's been discovered that the babybiome of the bundle of misery may be different from that of other babies. So it could be that unexplained screaming is a sign of *dysbiosis* (if you remember from Chapter 2, that's when the gut bugs are out of whack).

While the idea that colic could be a bug problem is far from clear, here's what we know so far:

- The colic babybiome is less diverse than "normal" babies.
- Screamers have fewer good bacteria, like the *Bifido* and *Lactobacillus* species, and more *Proteobacteria,* which are less healthy and can cause gas.
- The colic babybiome is more like that of a baby born by C-section or a baby fed artificial milk.

The babybiome and its relationship to behavior is a hot area of research, and our understanding of our bundles of misery will likely grow in the years ahead as a result of advancements in this space.

LACTOBACILLUS REUTERI: THE ANTICOLIC SUPERBUG

One of the most interesting bugs found to help the miserable baby is *Lactobacillus reuteri*. Studies comparing *L. reuteri* with simethicone, the secret weapon in gas drops, showed a significant reduction in crying in those babies given *L. reuteri*. Analysis of the stool of the treated babies demonstrated fewer gas-forming *E. coli,* which may explain some of the effect.

Premature babies given this interesting bug were found to have improvements in the way their stomachs emptied and moved. They also had fewer episodes of spitting. While we've always assumed that bacteria were hard at work in the colon, *L. reuteri* is one of the few bacteria found to colonize the entire baby gut, from upper intestine to colon. This impact on tummy squeezing may potentially explain some of the anticolic effects seen with strains like *L. reuteri*.

It's interesting to note that *L. reuteri* was isolated in 1990 from the breast milk of a Peruvian mother living in the Andes. This bug (along with many others) has been identified as an inhabitant of the breast duct and is likely part of what you deliver to your baby if breast-feeding. When we think about the amazing health benefits of breast milk, you have to wonder what role bacteria like *L. reuteri* play in conferring those benefits.

PROBIOTICS AND YOUR BABY'S HEALTH

W E OPENED *Looking Out for Number Two* WITH A DISCUSSION about the babybiome because so much of what's at the root of a baby's digestive health is the bacteria she carries. We learned that *how we deliver our babies* and *how we choose to feed* can impact the bugs our babies carry. And those bugs play a big role in shaping how healthy and immunologically competent our kids become.

But is there anything we can do to shift or tip the flora such that it works in our baby's favor?

As it turns out, there is. They're called *probiotics,* and if you've been paying attention, they're turning up in everyday foods from baby formula to yogurt drinks. But there's so much confusion about probiotics—do they actually do much or are they just a gimmick? Are they safe for babies? Do we use them to prevent or treat disease?

While this is a hot area of research that's continually developing, let's cover what we know and what you need to know about how probiotics support a healthy gut and a strong immune system, and how they can potentially benefit other parts of your baby's body as well.

PROBIOTIC BASICS

PROBIOTICS: BUGS WITH BENEFITS

If you have no idea what a probiotic is, you're in good company. You may be relieved (or shocked) to know that when I speak to groups of doctors and ask for a definition of probiotic, few are confident enough to stand up and define it.

Very simply, a probiotic is a living organism that, when ingested, has a positive impact on our health. To be a probiotic, it has to offer some kind of benefit—it has to do something for us or our baby. Many probiotic effects are not visible to the naked parental eye, but they have to be *functional* in a way that we can see through changes in diaper stuff or way down on the microscopic or molecular level.

When we talked about the billions of bugs in our baby, we discussed the idea of a *fingerprint*—a unique population of bacteria that inhabit the bowel and live in happy harmony. These balanced populations of bugs are important and many of these strains are actually probiotics. But as you've seen at various points in the book, the populations can get out of whack for any number of reasons. We can help things along by using probiotics to seed the bowel with bacteria that do very specific beneficial things. Probiotics are bugs with benefits.

If we agree that the trillions of bacteria that make up the babybiome constitute an actual organ, then think of probiotics as a targeted way to strengthen that organ and keep it ticking. And, in fact, we're approaching the point where healthy probiotic strains may not be optional for babies but rather represent a key nutritional element, like a beneficial food group.

HOW "GOOD BUGS" CAN MAKE YOUR BABY STRONGER AND HEALTHIER

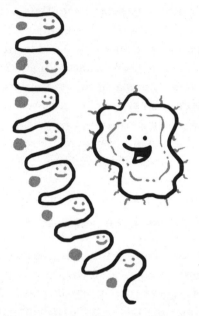

There are a lot of positive effects from probiotics. As we'll see, these effects vary from strain to strain, but in really general terms, we can think of probiotics as having a few key roles in promoting health in the gut and beyond:

- **Bacterial-immune cross-talk.** There's an ongoing dialogue between our probiotic bugs and our immune cells. Our immune system is typically primed to act and react, but probiotics serve as diplomats and help our immune system settle down and chill. When your baby's body "sees" bacteria, it is more at ease coexisting with them. Probiotics help the growing immune system begin to tell good from bad.

- **Occupy important real estate.** Remember that a gut lining has only so much landscape. Probiotics compete for that limited landscape in our gut and prevent the overgrowth of the bad guys. Think of probiotics as the police force of our bacterial flora.
- **Fortify the gut wall.** Beyond elbowing their way for a spot on the bowel wall, probiotic strains secure and fortify the intestinal barrier to keep it strong and intact so that other less-friendly things aren't causing problems by permeating the gut lining.
- **Simulate the immune system.** Beyond preventing pathogenic bacteria (the bad bacteria) from ever getting a leg up, probiotics trigger the immune system to create pathogen-zapping IgA, the first line of defense in fighting infection.

You can't see any of these effects, but the right strain in the right doses from the right source (food or supplement) will work its molecular magic behind the scenes.

There are some effects on things like viral diarrhea and colic that you can see with your eyes, and we'll get to those in a moment.

What's key is that when we study the many effects of probiotics, we see that they are supertargeted in their ability to do certain things well. As a result, talking about probiotics like they're all the same thing is quickly becoming a thing of the past.

WHY "TAKING A PROBIOTIC" MAY BE ON THE WAY OUT

It's a pretty regular conversation in my office: I'll talk with a mother who has come in for a specific problem, and she proudly tells me that she "just started probiotics last week." When I ask what strain, I get the probiotic deer-in-the-headlights look (that's the look from a mother when it's clear that she has absolutely no idea what she's giving her child or why).

Since the earliest days of probiotics, parents have jumped on board with the primitive idea that giving probiotics is good. And a lot like the whole organic food thing, we've seen a market explosion of products willing to fuel the craze for good bugs. But the reality is that just giving probiotics doesn't make much sense.

WE HAVE TO GIVE THE RIGHT PROBIOTIC FOR THE RIGHT REASON

Think about that UTI you had after you were pregnant. When you went to your OB, she didn't say, "we need to give you some antibiotics." Rather, she chose an antibiotic that's known to specifically target the bad bugs that we know live around your bottom. It wasn't just any old antibiotic, because if she chose the antibiotic that treats the stuff that grows on your skin, you would never have gotten better.

Antibiotics have to be targeted to suspect organisms. And this is the way that our thinking about probiotics is going as well. We're learning that certain strains are good at certain things, and that not all probiotics are created equal.

ARE PROBIOTICS SAFE FOR BABIES?

Before we get into specifics, let's address the elephant in the room: Are these things safe for babies?

When I speak to audiences of pediatricians about probiotics, I love to ask this question. Universally, every hand goes up to vote yes, they are safe. The rationale is that we give probiotics to babies all the time—in fact, we're finding them in infant formula. But it's a bit of a trick question, because the answer is that *it depends on the probiotic*. Staying true to the core idea that not all probiotics are created equal, we can't categorically say that *all* probiotics are safe for babies.

They have to be proven safe. And we can't say that about all strains. So let's explore how to use the right baby bugs for the right reasons.

WHERE DO BABIES GET PROBIOTICS

Speaking in general terms, we get probiotics from two sources: foods and supplements. Babies present a challenge on this first front, because their range of food sources are limited through much of the first year.

The best source of powerfully helpful probiotics is breast milk. As I've echoed throughout the book, if you have the choice about how to nourish your baby, breast milk should be your first choice for many reasons, but definitely for the bugs.

Other than breast milk and a few select foods late in the first year, we'll be dependent upon supplemental sources of probiotics for our babies' needs.

THE FAB FOUR | FUELING THE BABYBIOME WITH POWER STRAINS

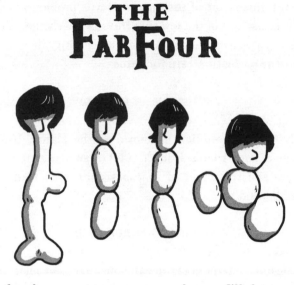

Rather than keep you in suspense any longer, I'll share my probiotic **Fab Four**. These are probiotic power strains for the growing baby. They have a long track record of safety and success, and they may have a role in helping keep your baby's biome in line. I'll do an introduction to the Fab Four first, and then I'll follow up with a few situations where you might be able to put them to use.

BIFIDOBACTERIA

Bifidobacteria is the mother of all probiotic strains and the gut bug of choice in breast-fed babies. When we look at what makes up the majority of the bowel flora in the breast-fed baby, this is it. While there's more that we don't know about this critter than we do know, it's clear that he's up to a whole lot of good.

LACTOBACILLUS REUTERI

Originally isolated from the breast ducts of a woman in the Peruvian Andes, this is one of the most versatile probiotic strains for babies. It is also one of the few that inhabit nearly the full length of the bowel, which means it has some interesting effects. *L. reuteri* is my favorite probiotic strain for babies.

LACTOBACILLUS GG (LGG)

Arguably the most studied probiotic on the planet, *LGG* is the workhorse of good bacteria. It has a lot of amazing effects in the prevention and treatment of diseases connected with the gut, skin, and beyond.

SACCHAROMYCES BOULARDII

This is the only organism of the Fab Four that's not a bacteria—it's actually a yeast. It does some wonderful things and should serve to remind us that the babybiome is made up of more than just bacteria (it also includes viruses and yeast).

CONDITIONS WHERE PROBIOTICS MAY PREVENT PROBLEMS OR FIX YOUR BABY

LET'S TALK ABOUT some cases where probiotics have been used to fix or prevent problems in babies. Remember that the media love to promote stories based on isolated one-off studies. So while probiotics may be suggested to help in a variety of situations, we'll stick to some of the more established problems where therapeutic bugs show promise.

COLIC—A DISEASE OF DYSBIOSIS?

We've already learned that colic is a wastebasket diagnosis used when pediatricians are outwitted or just plain out of ideas. As it turns out, some studies support the idea that the bundle of misery has a different pattern of bacteria in the colon. One of the big differences reported in colicky babies is a relative shortage of *lactobacilli* organisms.

The connection between different intestinal bacteria and the risk for profound fussiness is unclear, although it could be connected to the fact that a healthy population of bacteria help establish a strong gut barrier that keeps things that don't belong from getting into the blood.

Irrespective of why, clinical studies have demonstrated marked improvement in colic symptoms with the use of the probiotic strain *L. reuteri*. When compared against babies treated with simethicone (the active ingredient in many gas drops), the amount of time spent crying among babies treated with *L. reuteri* was markedly less. Follow-up studies have demonstrated that *L. reuteri* has a specific antimicrobial effect against six species of gas-forming colon bugs. It's worth noting that while the mechanism of cutting colic in babies isn't exactly clear, children with abdominal pain have been shown to report decreased intensity of their pain with this bug. It's clear that something good is going on.

This colic result showcases the key fact that certain probiotic strains work for certain things. As it turns out, *L. reuteri* is the only organism that has demonstrated an improvement in colic symptoms in babies. It's also important to remember that babies cry for a lot of reasons beyond bacteria. We've got to keep our eyes and ears open to other treatable conditions, like allergy and reflux.

DIARRHEA

Not many things are more miserable than diarrhea in a baby. And beyond the misery of a broken-down bottom is the real risk of dehydration—diarrhea needs to be taken seriously, since little people can get dry really fast. See Chapter 4 for more details.

There is evidence in otherwise healthy babies to support the use of probiotics early in the course of diarrhea from viruses. Studies show that probiotic strains such as *Lactobacillus GG* and *S. boulardii* reduce the duration of diarrhea by about a day.

Prevention of diarrhea may be another story. Studies don't yet support the routine use of probiotics to *prevent* infectious diarrhea in babies, though some studies show a benefit with use of probiotics such as *LGG* and *S. boulardii* to prevent antibiotic-associated diarrhea.

Keep in mind that while we may not offer a daily probiotic such as *LGG* to a baby strictly to prevent the diarrhea that may result from a day-care setting, benefits to the babybiome and beyond may make it a solid choice for your baby and her budding immune system.

ECZEMA AND ALLERGIES

Throughout *Looking Out for Number Two,* there's been a lot of mention of the connection between the bugs our babies bear and intestinal issues.

But remember that bacteria are in constant conversation with all the immune cells living around the gut (70 percent of a baby's immune cells are situated there). Those cells migrate and impact the health of other organs, like the skin (yes, the skin is an organ) and the lungs. The connection between the gut and the skin and lungs is often forgotten, but these organs feel the full force of a hyperactive or inexperienced immune system.

As it turns out, the bugs found in children with eczema and allergies are very different from those of children without eczema. Kids with eczema and allergies have more *Clostridium* bugs and fewer *Bifidobacterium* organisms than children without eczema. This has led doctors to consider using probiotics in kids at risk for diseases like eczema.

Studies have shown that *Lactobacillus GG* (*LGG*) given to mothers during the last trimester of pregnancy and while breast-feeding during the first six months of life reduces the incidence of eczema in at-risk babies.

Although evidence to date has suggested a potential preventative role for certain probiotics in eczema, there is no evidence to support that probiotics actually treat it once it's fully blossomed.

REFLUX

Whoa, wait . . . probiotics for reflux?

Remember how *L. reuteri* is one of the few bugs that lives top to bottom in the gut? It turns out that babies with reflux showed improvement in tummy squeezing and reflux when treated with *L. reuteri*. While studies to date on *L. reuteri* and reflux have been interesting, it isn't standard treatment to use probiotic bugs for baby heartburn—yet. Stay tuned.

PROBIOTICS AS PREVENTION OR REACTION

Not long ago during a trip overseas, I had the pleasure of having dinner with three pediatricians from Sweden. Over the course of our visit we shared experiences with how and when we use probiotics in babies. What became clear really quickly is the difference in mind-set between American and European doctors: in Europe, probiotics are seen to *prevent* disease, while in the United States, probiotics are used to *treat* disease. We wait until people get sick and then react to it, but our neighbors across the pond see things differently.

You'll probably see this bias reflected in your discussions with your pediatrician. He or she will likely recommend specific probiotics to make bad things go away. But as a profession, American pediatricians are not at the point where they routinely recommend probiotics for babies as a means of preventing disease. I suspect that the growing body of research will evolve to change U.S. practice to be more in line with that of our European neighbors.

I RECOMMEND BABIES GET ONE OF THE FAB FOUR

With that said, I'm a strong believer in the power and potential of healthy bugs. Given the cellular impact of healthy bacterial strains on the gut and immune system, I don't see how we can deny babies this opportunity. Evidence is mounting that probiotic prevention trumps treatment, so I encourage routine use of one of the Fab Four during the formative fourth trimester of gut and immune development. I favor *L. reuteri* and *LGG* as solid prophylactic probiotics early in childhood.

BREAST-FEEDING WILL GIVE YOUR BABY BUGS, BUT NOT QUITE ENOUGH

While breast-feeding is the optimal power fuel for your baby, the numbers of bugs she'll get may not be enough for maximal impact. Breast or bottle, I advocate supplementation.

GRANDPA JERRY'S URN

You could say that probiotics are in my blood. When my grandfather immigrated from Armenia in 1913, he brought with him two things through Ellis Island: his little sister and a vial of starter culture for his yogurt. He knew that active, probiotic cultures were critical to survival in the new world. So faith in probiotics runs in my family. I suspect, however, that if Grandpa Jerry were here, he would probably laugh at our science and preach the power of a healthy, balanced Mediterranean-type diet consisting of fresh, whole foods with natural sources of active cultures. And I can't say I would disagree!

PRACTICAL ISSUES OF GIVING A PROBIOTIC TO A BABY

HOW EARLY CAN YOU GIVE YOUR BABY A PROBIOTIC?

Babies can receive certain probiotics starting in their earliest days. In fact, certain probiotic species are used in some neonatal intensive care units as a means of preventing necrotizing enterocolitis, a dangerous bowel condition prevalent among preemies. Remember too that babies are exposed to many species of probiotic bacteria through breast milk. Probiotics have been in infant formula for many years in Europe and, more recently, in the United States.

IS THERE EVER A TIME WHEN YOU SHOULDN'T USE A PROBIOTIC IN A BABY?

If your baby is anything other than a happy, healthy, bouncing baby, you should use probiotics (or any supplement, for that matter) only in close cooperation with your health-care provider. The American Academy of Pediatrics has suggested that probiotics or formulas containing probiotics *should not be given to seriously ill children or those with immune problems*.

TIPS FOR GIVING YOUR BABY A POWDERED PROBIOTIC

Since babies don't take capsules and can't yet eat foods that naturally contain probiotic strains, you'll be limited to powders and drops. Drops can typically be put directly into your baby's mouth. If you're giving a powder, moisten a finger and create a coating with the probiotic powder, then make a sweep into your baby's mouth. Powder can also be applied directly to your breast before and during feeding.

Add probiotic powder or drops to a bottle only as a last resort. If your baby doesn't complete her bottle, she doesn't complete her bugs. Add it to the smallest volume of formula or expressed breast milk that you know she'll complete.

SHOULD YOU USE AN INFANT FORMULA WITH ADDED PROBIOTIC?

It wasn't that long ago that we were preoccupied with the purity of our baby's milk. Sterilization and purity have given way to the idea that bacteria may have a home in our baby's formula. In 2008, the first probiotic supplemented infant formula was approved by the FDA (*Bifidobacteria* in Nestlé Good Start with Natural Cultures), and in 2009 Mead Johnson followed suit (*Lactobacillus GG* in Nutramigen). In addition to these two formulas, Nestlé introduced Nestlé Good Start Soothe, which contains my favorite bug, *L. reuteri.*

So if you can't breast-feed and have to use formula, you can avoid supplementation by using a milk with bugs built right in. The only downside here is that probiotic formulas are limited to powdered forms in order to avoid the heat treatment that liquid formulas have to go through (as this would kill the bacteria).

BEYOND MILK AND SUPPLEMENTS | THE PROBIOTIC SHOPPING CART

THE TWO PHASES during a baby's first year for seeding and fueling a healthy babybiome are before solids and after solids. Before you start giving your baby food, her only source of probiotics is milk and supplements. After starting solids, her world will begin to open up to more natural sources of bugs.

While supplements are fine, some evidence suggests that we're better off getting our bacteria from food rather than drops. One of the obstacles to getting the right number of bacteria into our colon is survival of the bugs during their miraculous journey through the intestinal system. The acidic environment of the stomach is troublesome for bacteria, and live bacteria tend to survive better when their journey is cushioned and buffered by food.

So the bottom line is that once your baby has started solids, food is a better source of bugs than drops and powders.

WHERE DO YOU FIND GOOD BACTERIA IN A BABY'S DIET?

Although lots of foods contain healthy active bacteria cultures (sauerkraut, poi, tempeh, sourdough bread), most babies aren't self-feeding sauerkraut before their first birthday . . . or their second. Until then, leverage the probiotic power foods like yogurt and soft cheeses.

WHEN CAN YOU GIVE A BABY YOGURT AND CHEESE?

I hopefully made it clear in Chapter 3 that milk in liquid form is something we hold until a baby hits her first birthday. But that doesn't mean that babies can't be exposed to things with milk. Yogurt and cheese are cultured milk products that are fine to give to a baby under a year, though we have to be careful about how much we offer. I typically allow babies to have yogurt after eight months of age and in amounts limited to about four ounces. Cheese fits into this same category of milk product, so it should be included in those total four ounces as well. This four-ounce rule is just an approximation, but it helps provide a general guideline for parents.

YOGURT IS NOT EXACTLY MEDICINE

Parents like to give their children yogurt when they are sick or on antibiotics. While I love the concept of food as medicine, the job of fixing an obliterated babybiome may not be as simple as it looks.

As our understanding of the microbiome has evolved, we've learned that you need to take in substantial numbers of organisms to treat disease. And what we get in a container of yogurt isn't likely to be a medicinal quantity.

Consider what we find in our friendly neighborhood yogurt tub:

Yogurt source	Serving	Probiotic serving
Yogurt with live bacteria	6–8 ounces	6–20 billion bacteria
Frozen yogurt with bacteria	4 ounces	1–3 billion bacteria
Probiotic shots	3–4 ounces	6–20 billion bacteria
Kefir	8 ounces	3–10 billion bacteria

This table is modified from *The Probiotics Revolution* by Gary Huffnagle, PhD.

Now consider that it takes on the order of twenty billion bugs to treat the diarrhea associated with antibiotics. You're looking at more high-quality yogurt than most babies and toddlers are able or willing to consume. As another example of how high we sometimes need to go, we're using around 450 billion bacteria when we use probiotics to treat ulcerative colitis in older children.

So food as medicine is very different from food that creates healthy balance. In the end, a healthy balanced diet rich in active cultures will serve to keep your baby healthy rather than pull them back from the brink once you're facing dangerous dysbiosis.

A FEW KEY POINTS ON CHOOSING YOGURT FOR YOUR BABY

The kind of yogurt you offer your baby is important especially when you consider the amount of sugar commonly found in some of the popular brands.

MAKE SURE IT ACTUALLY HAS BUGS

Yogurt is in the eye of the beholder, or manufacturer. Never assume that just because it is called yogurt that it carries any real nutritional value.

Look for products with the "Live and Active Cultures" seal from the National Yogurt Association. It's important to note that the milk is pasteurized *before* culturing to remove any harmful bacteria. Some yogurts are heated after fermentation, which kills most of the beneficial active cultures found in the yogurt.

YOGURT AND CANDY YOGURT

Yogurt packaged and marketed to children can be high in sugar. For example, six ounces of Danimals brand yogurt contains approximately twenty grams of sugar. Compare that to an equivalent volume of Coca-Cola, which contains nineteen grams of sugar. Yes, you read that correctly.

Beyond wreaking havoc with children's metabolism, foods with high sugar quantities sets expectations about how our food is supposed to taste. Once you develop a tongue for the sweet stuff, it's hard to go back.

ACTIVE CULTURES ARE BITTER

All this added sugar results from the fact that yogurt is inherently bitter. Active cultures can give kids serious bitter face, and a small amount of sweet stuff can offset the negative reaction. This sweet-and-bitter balance is a trade-off we face with kids and yogurt.

WHEN LIFE GIVES YOU BABY POO, MAKE SAUSAGE
Spanish researchers have determined that one of the most powerful bacterial cultures for the production of fermented sausage comes from baby poo. In a paper published in 2015 entitled "Characterization of Lactic Acid Bacteria Isolated from Infant Faeces as

Potential Probiotic Starter Cultures for Fermented Sausages," researchers showcase the power of what you find on the operating end of a baby wipe (and might make you think twice about ordering sausage in Madrid).

SAVING POO FOR A RAINY DAY

While we parents traditionally have encouraged our children to save money, it seems that there may be a movement to save our poo. With rising interest in the microbiota and everything that goes with it, businesses have emerged that allow you to store, or "bank," your healthy bugs in the event that you need to repopulate your gut with the good guys. While I've yet to hear of mothers banking diaper sausages, it does give new meaning to "investing for their future."

Thoughts on the Future
of Parents and Poo

WHO KNEW THAT SOMEONE COULD ACTUALLY WRITE A WHOLE BOOK on baby poo? I did, and it's been a blast. But this is really just a start. Everything we understand about the role of nutrition, poo, and the babybiome is just beginning to come to the forefront.

In the early 1990s, I remember seeing patients with Texas Children's Hospital's Dr. William Klish, one of the founders of the field of pediatric gastroenterology. He was one of the first professionals to identify the parental preoccupation with poo. In fact, he was the first person I heard characterize the curious chroniclers of diaper patterns as stool gazers. On a certain level we saw it as amusing at the time. It was tongue-in-cheek. But I've come to see that the observing parents we looked after were ahead of even this brilliant pioneer of pediatric digestive health.

Over the twenty-five years since Dr. Klish introduced me to the concept, I have come to respect the wisdom of the parents who bring their stories, pictures, spreadsheets, and concerns about poo. It's these details and descriptions, coupled with the clear emerging power of the babybiome, that tell me that we're on to something when we pay attention to parents and their tales of poo. What babies do or don't do, and how poo smells, looks, or emerges from the colon, tells us so much about the well-being of a young person. As suggested at the outset of *Number Two,* I suspect the future will prove that your baby's diaper is the window to her soul.

But we've just begun to scratch the surface of our understanding of how the gut sets a baby up for a long, healthy life. I predict that during the lifetime of the baby you now hold, everything we understand about how to feed and care for babies with respect to gut health will be turned upside down. In fact, it's already started. So don't be afraid to ask the crazy questions. Remember that it wasn't long ago that we were engaged in war with any microbe that came within arm's reach of the baby in our arms. Now we recognize that bacteria are an integral part of breast milk, and we even put them into infant formula.

Hopefully, *Looking Out for Number Two* has offered a primer on how to think about your baby from the inside out. While poo is an afterthought for many parents, my hope is that you've come to respect the importance of the first months, days, and even hours of life with respect to how babies are nourished and exposed to the world. More than fixing all your poo problems, I would like to think that I've given you the firepower and confidence to start a conversation between you and your mother-in-law, friends, or pediatrician. I hope you've found this empowering.

As twentieth-century parenting mogul Benjamin Spock suggested, you know more than you think you do. So don't be afraid to speak up and show us what your baby is making. Her life may depend upon it.

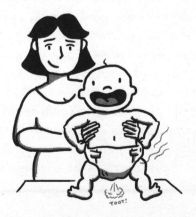

ACKNOWLEDGMENTS

THEY SAY THAT BOOKS ON POO TAKE A VILLAGE. I WANT TO THANK Sarah Murphy at Harper Wave who saw the potential of *Number Two* and was an absolute pleasure to work with. This never would have seen the light of day without the insight and wisdom of Jessica Papin at Dystel and Goderich Literary Management.

RDNs Kristi King, Lauren Manaker, and Jamie Bocella offered a dietitian's critical eye. Drs. Tony Olive, Bruno Chumpitazi, Bill Klish, Carla Davis, Susie O'Neal, Charles Hankins, Maureen Leonard, and Michelle Pietzak offered critical input on different parts of the manuscript. I will add that any final copy irregularities related to my hard-nosed view of digestive health are my responsibility alone. It should be noted that my thinking about digestive health is only possible because of the daily input of my colleagues in the Division of Pediatric Gastroenterology at Texas Children's Hospital in Houston and Texas Children's Hospital | The Woodlands. It's an honor to work in America's greatest children's hospital.

I want to thank Zach Harris of BirdsandKings.com for his brilliant and spot-on illustrations. A nod to Mike Rohde who graciously connected me to Zach.

As always, none of what I do would be possible without my wife Deidre and my children Laura and Nick, who selflessly allow me the space and time to think and create.

Index

ABOUT THE AUTHOR

BRYAN VARTABEDIAN IS A PEDIATRIC GASTROENTEROLOGIST AT TEXAS Children's Hospital in Houston, America's largest children's hospital. Beyond examining thousands of dirty diapers, he has made a life shaping practical solutions to the digestive health problems of children. He is the author of *Colic Solved*, and he lives in The Woodlands, Texas with his wife, two children, and an Australian labradoodle.